THE AGONY ABIDES

THE AGONY ABIDES

An Anthology

compiled by

Bronwen Wrigley

WAVENEY

First published in 2010 by Waveney
94 Riverside Drive, Stoneclough, Radcliffe, Manchester, M26 1HY

Distributed by Gardners Books
1 Whittle Drive, Eastbourne, East Sussex, BN23 6QH
Tel: +44(0)1323 521555 | Fax: +44(0)1323 521666

British Library Cataloguing in Publication Data
A catalogue record for this book is available from the British Library

ISBN 978-0-9562772-0-6

Typeset by Amolibros, Milverton, Somerset
www.amolibros.com
This book production has been managed by Amolibros
Printed and bound by T J International Ltd, Padstow, Cornwall, UK

Dedicated to Lyndon with much love and many thanks

CONTENTS

Preface

> "Until...man finds evil unmistakably present in his existence, in the form of pain, he is enclosed in illusion. Once pain has roused him, he knows he is in some way or other, 'up against' the real universe."[1]

This is not a book about depression. It contains no tips on how to 'banish the blues' nor does it offer suggestions as to the best types of therapy to try. Rather, in compiling *The Agony Abides* I have attempted to convey a fundamental truth; one that is becoming increasingly difficult to hear in a society ever more dependent on inanity, trivia and shallowness.

This truth is that far from being the party our modern age promises, life is a very serious thing indeed, and if faced up to realistically is, to quote C S Lewis, "unbearable". Unfortunately, few people do face up to it realistically, preferring instead to live in a permanent Disneyland. So wedded now is our culture to humanistic ideology with its emphasis on positive thinking, progress and optimism, that anyone who confronts the dismal truth about life, and suffers emotionally as a result, is judged as being 'disturbed' and in need of 'help'.

The late Erich Fromm, an eminent German psychiatrist, believed that in actual fact the opposite is true. He argued that it is usually the people whom society labels disturbed or neurotic who are in fact the ones most sane and alive, observing that there is always hope for such people, despite the anguish and despair they experience, because they are reacting as healthy people should react to the horrors of life, whereas those whom society considers 'normal' are actually the hopeless victims.

"Many of them are normal," Fromm says, "because they are so well adjusted to our mode of existence, [and] because their human voice has been silenced so early in their lives that they do not...struggle or suffer or develop symptoms as the neurotic does."[2]

I am a person who has long been labelled 'neurotic' and in need of treatment by 'normal' people. One of the purposes of *The Agony Abides* is an attempt to defend my deeply held belief that low spirits, sadness and melancholy are not symptoms of a disease from which we need to be cured, but rather are the correct and rational responses of thinking human beings to life in a fallen world.

Another reason why I have compiled the anthology is that I believe there is much purpose served in reading about the distress of others. As Charlotte Bronte wrote:

> "If we ourselves live in fullness of content, it is well to be reminded that thousands of our fellow creatures undergo a different lot.... If, on the other hand, we be contending with the special grief, the intimate trial, the peculiar bitterness with which God has seen fit to mingle our own cup of existence, it is very good to know that our overcast lot is not singular..."

My main reason, however, for compiling *The Agony Abides* is that I hope it will help those people who feel anomalous; 'different' from the average person. Often solitary, serious and introspective, those of a melancholic disposition are beset by an innate sorrow that is ever-present, a kind of sorrow that is increasingly misunderstood in these modern times. Surrounded by experts on every side, who tell us what to say, what to think, how to behave, how to feel; unable to escape the media's intrusive presence that forces on us a world with

That is the purpose of my anthology – to offer a collection of quotations for the 'unfortunate few' – those people of usually above-average intelligence who understand the meaning of life in a way that the more ordinary person does not. It is my hope that by reading passages written by others of melancholic disposition, readers may find some consolation - even if only, ironically, by discovering that there IS no consolation!

I close with a short quotation from Thompson's 'The City of Dreadful Night,' an utterly bleak poem that sums up the essence of what I hope this anthology will achieve.

This life holds nothing good for us
But it ends soon and never more can be.
I ponder these thoughts and they comfort me.

Notes

1. All Psalms and most other biblical passages are from the *King James Bible* (*Authorised Version*) or the *Book of Common Prayer*. However, excerpts from the Book of Job are from the *New International Version*. Although I do not generally like this translation, I think the meaning of the Job passages needs to be quite clear to be effective.

2. I have included a number of my own poems, all haikus. A haiku is a tiny poem originating in Japan, which traditionally has three unrhymed lines of, respectively, five, seven and five syllables, though this can vary slightly. I had never written a haiku before the terrible night in January 1999, when I sat up alone till after four a.m. and composed these somewhat clumsy attempts, knowing that the next day, when I went to see a diagnostician, he would tell me I was suffering from MS, the disease I had lived in dread of since my mother had been afflicted with it twenty years earlier (he did).

A haiku is meant to represent just one central idea, which must be clear, yet profound enough to stimulate thought, and that is what I tried to do. Each poem is meant to be complete in itself, yet is also linked to the others – like petals on a single flower.

In a way, all the writings I have chosen in this anthology are similar to haikus. Their themes are all distinct, like separate petals, yet they all make up one idea, one message. This message is, to quote Tolstoy, that "life is a cruel and stupid cheat".

Nothing lasts. Even the good things are marred. Everything is taken from us, and so on...

3. Some of the chapters are much longer than others, and also, some contain more of one type of passage. This is because certain themes are more commonly represented by a particular kind of quotation – for instance, the theme on fading loves has a larger amount of song lyrics than does that on the fear of death, which contains far more philosophical prose passages than song lyrics.

4. I had originally intended to arrange the passages thematically - ie, to enter them under a heading such as 'Youth and Age', 'The Fear of Death' and so on. However, as many of the quotations did not fit into a tightly structured theme (and conversely, some could have been included in several), I realised that it was impossible to do this.

I also did not want to strictly define the meaning of a passage, which the reader could interpret differently. Therefore, I have very loosely grouped the passages into chapters but rather than give a title to each one, I have instead begun the chapter with a quotation which gives a rough idea of what the passages will be 'about'. I hope that readers will find this way of arranging the material in the anthology more rewarding than a strict semantic/thematic structure would have been.

5. I believe that every passage in *The Agony Abides* contains some kind of deeply meaningful truth, and that long reflection is required in order for the meaning of the writings to be absorbed. Therefore, although the anthology can be read right through at one sitting (and perhaps that is the best way of approaching it initially), it will benefit most from careful, regular and thoughtful re-readings.

6. I have found it difficult to track down the copyright owners of every quotation, despite considerable efforts to find them. I apologise to any rights' holders for this. I also apologise for any errors which may feature in the anthology. The passages have been carefully checked and re-checked but it is not possible to guarantee total accuracy in the reproduction of other people's work.

Footnotes

1 C S Lewis, *The Problem of Pain*
2 Eric Fromm, *Brave New World Revisited* (Aldous Huxley)
3 Milan Kundera, *The Joke*
4 Oscar Wilde, *The Picture of Dorian Gray*
5 Voltaire, *Candide*
6 Malcolm Muggeridge, *Jesus Rediscovered*
7 Eric G Wilson, *Against Happiness: In Praise of Melancholy*
8 James Thompson, *The City of Dreadful Night*
9 Dick Sullivan, *Poison Mixed With Gall, The Victorian Web*

Anthology

Pain and fear, pain and fear for me, alive or dead.

Charles Dickens
Nicholas Nickleby

Years and infirmities oppress me, terror and anxiety beset me.

Samuel Johnson
Prayers and Meditations

Senseless and pointless worries occupy our minds.
Often our hearts, deprived of hope, are filled with fury.

John Mould
Motet 'Insanae Et Vanae Curae'

[W]hat no one ever dared think about the afterlife [is] that it might be exactly the same as this one.

Adam Phillips
Monogamy

Maybe the higher states of consciousness
Are other states of weariness

Emmett Tinley
Out of Mind

What is our life? A play of passion,
Our mirth the music of division…
Heaven the judicious sharp spector is
That sits and marks still who doth act amiss,
Our graves that hide us from the searching sun,
Are like drawn curtains when the play is done,
Thus march we playing to our latest rest,
Only we die in earnest, that's no jest.

Walter Raleigh
On the Life of Man

In the midst of life we are in death

Book of Common Prayer

Silent now, the lights
Are all gone out in the street
And I am afraid.

Bronwen Wrigley
Lifeless

Time rushes towards us with its hospital tray of infinitely varied narcotics, even while it is preparing us for its inevitably fatal operation.

Tennessee Williams
The Rose Tattoo

Alas! I have [not] hope nor health
Nor peace within nor calm around...
Nor fame nor power nor love nor leisure.
Others I see whom these surround –
Smiling they live and call life pleasure:
To me that cup has been dealt in another measure.

P B Shelley
Stanzas Written in Dejection Near Naples

Sometimes the strain falls on the mental, sometimes on the physical part of me; I am ill with headaches or I am ground to the dust with deep dejection of spirits.

Charlotte Bronte
The Life of Charlotte Bronte

"[I]s not the fear of death natural to man?"...
"So much so, Sir, that the whole of life is but keeping away the thoughts of it."

James Boswell/Samuel Johnson
The Life of Samuel Johnson

No one who has not known the unnameable torment involved in merely surviving the next ten seconds has any right to assume a lofty disdain of suicide.

Peter Mullen
Death be not Proud

Darker than night life's shadows fall around us,
And like benighted men we miss our mark:
God hides Himself, and grace hath scarcely found us,
E'er death finds out his victims in the dark.

Frederick W Faber
Hark Hark My Soul

The weariest and most loathed worldly life
That age, ache, penury and imprisonment
Can lay on nature, is a paradise
To what we fear of death.

William Shakespeare
Measure to Measure

My heart is disquieted within me: and the fear of death is fallen upon me.
Fearfulness and trembling are come upon me: and an horrible dread hath overwhelmed me.

Psalm 55

But better down there in the battle
Than here on the hill
With Judgement or nothingness waiting me
Lonely and chill.

John Betjeman
Goodbye

Is there anything on earth which cannot be doubted except death, the only certainty in this world?

E M Cioran
On the Heights of Despair

Nothing looks the same
Even my home is deformed
And everything changed.

Bronwen Wrigley
Illness

We decay,
Like corpses in a charnel; fear and grief
Convulse us and consume us day by day,
And cold hopes swarm like worms within our living clay.

P B Shelley
Adonais

I no longer sleep...and the little rest I get is broken by bad dreams...and fear. Atrocious fear presses me down, holds me without respite, never lets me go. Where is the justice in it all? What have I done to deserve this excess of severity?

Roubinovitch
La Melancolie

Who would bear the whips and scorns of time
But that dread of something after death,
The undiscover'd country from whose bourn
No traveller returns – puzzles the will
And makes us rather bear the ills we have
Than fly to others that we know not of?

William Shakespeare
Hamlet

When we reflect deeply on how life really is, both inside our soul and outside in our world, a quiet terror threatens to overwhelm us.

Larry Crabb
Inside Out

Waking at four to soundless dark, I stare
In time the curtain edges will grow light.
Till then I see what's really always there:
Unresting death, a whole day nearer now.

Philip Larkin
Aubade

Awake [or] asleep, the same thoughts lived in his brain. Frustration and bereavement...Failure and loss...Was all...joy gone [for ever]? Perhaps not, but it would have changed its tone, and would be edged with memories. And his own life; what did [that] add up to?...[A] part of his life was ended... a phase, an epoch, a turning...What had ended with this phase? Was it his youth? [And] [h]ow would he feel tonight if everything had happened different[ly] – if he...was not bereaved and beaten, light-headed and tired to death? He would have been asleep and safe from these thoughts. Yet would the phase have ended just the same? He did not know, and was too down to care. It did not seem just then that success in anything had ever been possible or that anything would ever be possible again. Failure was the end of life, all effort was dust, necessary and complete. All roads led to the bleak parapet of death.

Winston Graham
Demelza

I sleep not day nor night. Why is none of the heaviness of my heart dispensed into mine eyelids?

John Donne
Devotions

My apprehensions come in crowds,
I dread the rustling of the grass,
The very shadows of the clouds
Have power to shake me as they pass.
I question things and do not find
One that will answer to my mind
And all the world appears unkind.

William Wordsworth
The Affliction of Margaret

What I feared has come upon me
What I dreaded has happened to me
I have no peace, no quietness
I have no rest, but only turmoil.

Book of Job

Will I remember
The last night of my life
As a girl without MS?

Bronwen Wrigley
Terror

The sharpness of our perception of the world, the depth of our feelings about it, coupled with the knowledge of our own finiteness: these things add to the melancholy power of death.

Peter Mullen
Death be not Proud

As he passed through the fields he saw the animals around him. "Ye" said he, "are happy, and need not envy me that walk thus among you, burthened with myself. I have many distresses from which ye are free; I fear pain when I do not feel it; I sometimes shrink at evils recollected, and sometimes start at evils anticipated."

Samuel Johnson
The History of Rasselas

[T]he threat of death is...linked to a whole series of other conditions that...threaten to drain even the days we have left of meaning and purpose.

Joshua Foa Dienstag
Pessimism

You know how it is sometimes,
Some days you just wake up terrified?

Lyndon Morgans
She Lets Me in by the Back Door

I must write one line out of my weary bed. Let me speak plain truth – my sufferings are very great – my nights indescribable; sickness with scarce a reprieve.

Charlotte Bronte
The Life of Charlotte Bronte

I see
The lost are like this, and their scourge to be
As I am mine, their sweating selves; but worse.

Gerard Manley Hopkins
I Wake and Feel the Fell Of Dark

Put me not to rebuke, O Lord, in thine anger: neither chasten me in thy heavy displeasure. For thy arrows stick fast in me: and thy hand presseth me sore. There is no health in my flesh, because of thy displeasure: neither is there any rest in my bones, by reason of my sin. For my wickednesses are gone over my head: and are like a sore burden, too heavy for me to bear. I am brought into so great trouble and misery: that I go mourning all the day long. For my loins are filled with a sore disease: and there is no whole part in my body.

Psalm 38

Only the child who somewhere feels safe can take risks. Adults are [far] less daring than children because they...never feel safe.

Adam Phillips
Monogamy

The monotony of her life returned upon her in all its force; the only events of her days and weeks consisting in the small changes which occasional letters brought. Her health was such as to prevent her stirring out of the house. Sleeplessness, loss of appetite and continual headaches had brought her to a pitch of dangerous weakness. With illness came the old heaviness of heart, recollections of the past and anticipations of the future. Depression and solitude lay on her spirits like a pall.

Margaret Lane
The Bronte Story

In the languor of disease how little can be done.

Samuel Johnson
Letter to Mr Windham

The last year's leaves are on the beech:
The twigs are black; the cold is dry;
To deeps beyond the deepest reach
The Easter bells enlarge the sky.
Oh! Ordered metal clatter-clang!
Is yours the song the angels sang?
You fill my heart with joy and grief –
Belief! Belief! And unbelief...
And, though you tell me I shall die,
You say not how or when or why.
Indifferent the finches sing,
Unheeding roll the lorries past:
What misery will this year bring
Now spring is in the air at last?
For, sure as blackthorn bursts to snow,
Cancer in some of us will grow,
The tasteful crematorium door
Shuts out for some the furnace roar;
But church-bells open on the blast
Our loneliness, so long and vast.

John Betjeman
Loneliness

It feels like Christmas Eve,
Up so late, the house so quiet.
How wrong can you be?

Bronwen Wrigley
Delusion

We do not have to visit a madhouse to find disordered minds; our planet is the mental institution of the universe.

J W Von Goethe
Sensible Sayings

The reality of the body is one of the most terrible realities.

E M Cioran
On the Heights of Despair

In the name of Hypocrites, doctors have invented the most exquisite form of torture ever known
to man: survival.

Luis Bunuel
My Last Sigh

That which is living…[c]an only die.

T S Eliot
Four Quartets (Burnt Norton)

There is a special way of being afraid
No trick dispels. Religion used to try,
That vast moth-eaten musical brocade
Created to pretend we never die…
Most things may never happen: this one will,
And realisation of it rages out
In furnace fear when we are caught without
People or drink.

Philip Larkin
Audabe

Boswell writes about the difficult fact that people will still be young and flowers will still bloom when we are dead, and the last pages of his book are almost choked with sickness, melancholy
and death.

Angus Calder
Introduction to the Life of Samuel Johnson

The oppression of frequent headaches, sickness and a low tone of spirits has poisoned many moments which might otherwise have been pleasant.

Charlotte Bronte
The Life of Charlotte Bronte

What on earth was all the fun for?
For I'm old and ill and terrified.

John Betjeman
Sun and Fun

I knew I would never walk
The Pennine Way. I did not think
That I would never walk.

Bronwen Wrigley
Pennine Way

All natural happiness seems infected with a contradiction. The breath of the sepulchre surrounds it. Our troubles lie indeed too deep for any cure. The fact that we *can* die, that we *can* be ill at all, is what perplexes us; the fact that we now for a moment live and are well is irrelevant to that perplexity. We need a life not correlated with death, a health not liable to illness, a kind of good that will not perish.

William James
The Varieties of Religious Experience

Once again, sleepless and empty

Emmett Tinley
Love and Possession

Of my health I cannot tell you…that it is much improved by the season or by remedies. I am sleepless; my legs grow weary with a very few steps. Nights of watchfulness produce torpid days; I read very little though I am alone. This is my history, like all other histories – a narrative of misery.

Samuel Johnson
Letter to Mr Windham

I dare say I shall be glad sometime, but I am so ill, so weary

Charlotte Bronte
The Life of Charlotte Bronte

He hath…brought me into darkness, but not into light.

Lamentations 3

Kind people have said to me, "She is with God…she is in God's hands." But if so, she was in God's hands all the time, and I have seen what they did to her here. Do they suddenly become gentler to us the moment we are out of the body? And if so, why? If God's goodness is inconsistent with hurting us, then either God is not good or there is no God: for in the only life we know He hurts us beyond our worst fears and beyond all we can imagine. If it is consistent with hurting us, then He may hurt us after death as unendurably as before it.

C S Lewis
A Grief Observed

Nay, but for terror of his wrathful face
I swear I will not call injustice 'Grace'.

Edward Fitzgerald
Rubaiyat of Omar Khayyam

Just for a change, God
Leaves us alone, sits back and
Counts the fallen sparrows.[9]

Bronwen Wrigley
Respite

Have mercy upon me, O Lord, for I am weak:
O Lord, heal me, for my bones are vexed.
My soul also is sore troubled: but Lord, how long wilt thou punish me?

Psalm 6

God gives nuts to those with no teeth.

Anon
Arabic Proverb

The strongest case against God comes…from the billions of normal lives that are full of apparently pointless suffering. It is not just that suffering is not deserved; it is that it seems so random…distributed according to no rhyme or reason but mere chance, and working no good in the end. For every one who becomes a hero and a saint through suffering, there are ten who… become dehumanised, depressed, or despairing.

Peter Kreeft
Making Sense Out of Suffering

Only grant me these two things, Oh God
Withdraw your hand from me
And stop frightening me with your terrors.

Book of Job

What Power delights to torture us? I know
That to myself I do not wholly owe
What now I suffer, though in part I may.
Alas, none strewed sweet flowers upon the way

P B Shelley
A Conversation

From my youth I have been afflicted and close to death;
I have suffered your terrors and am in despair.
Your wrath has swept over me;
Your terrors have destroyed me
The darkness is my closest friend.

Psalm 88

Comforter, where, where is your comforting?
Mary, mother of us, where is your relief?

Gerard Manley Hopkins
No Worst, There is None

But go to Him when your need is desperate, when all other help is vain, and what do you find? A door slammed in your face, and a sound of bolting and double bolting on the inside. After that, silence. You may as well turn away. The longer you wait, the more emphatic the silence will become.

Not that I am (I think) in much danger of ceasing to believe in God. The real danger is in coming to believe such dreadful things about Him. The conclusion I dread is not, "So there's no God at all", but, "So this is what God's really like. Deceive yourself no longer".

C S Lewis
A Grief Observed

We are no other than a moving row
Of magic shadow shapes that come and go
Round with the sun-illumined lantern held
In midnight by the Master of the show.

But helpless pieces of the game he plays
Upon this chequerboard of nights and days
Hither and thither moves, and checks, and slays
And one by one back in the closet lays.

Edward Fitzgerald
Rubaiyat of Omar Khayyam

For these things I weep; mine eye runneth down with water, because the comforter that should relieve my soul is far from me.

Lamentations 1

When I think my bed will comfort me, even then you frighten me with dreams. Let me alone.

Book of Job

And where will you be
When they wheel me on the trolley
Down the endless corridor?

Bronwen Wrigley
Jesus

One day when God says He wishes things had been different
I'll say, "Mmm, me too..."

Lyndon Morgans
One Day When God Begs My Forgiveness

My soul is full of trouble: and my life draweth nigh unto hell...
Thou hast laid me in the lowest pit: in a place of darkness, and in the deep.
Thine indignation lieth hard upon me: and thou hast vexed me with all thy storms.
Thou hast put away mine acquaintance far from me: and made me to be abhorred of them.
I am so fast in prison: that I cannot get forth.
My sight faileth for very trouble: Lord, I have called daily upon thee, I have stretched forth my hands unto thee...
Lord, why abhorrest thou my soul: and hidest thou thy face from me?

Psalm 88

What chokes every prayer and every hope is the memory of all the prayers we offered and all the false hopes we had. Not hopes raised merely by our own wishful thinking. Step by step we were 'led up the garden path'. Time after time, when He seemed most gracious He was really preparing the next torture.

C S Lewis
A Grief Observed

Surely, Oh God, you have worn me out...

Book of Job

Age, I do abhor thee.

William Shakespeare
A Madrigal

I tell you kid it's tough, best you don't ever grow up.

Lyndon Morgans
Just Another Night in Limbo

The first half of life consists of the capacity to enjoy without the chance; the last half consists of the chance without the capacity.

Mark Twain
Mark Twain's Philosophy on Life

This breathing house not built with hands,
This body that does me grievous wrong,
O'er aery cliffs and glittering sands,
How lightly then it flashed along-
Like those trim skiffs, unknown of yore,
On winding lakes and rivers wide,
That ask no aid of sail or oar,
That fear no spite of wind or tide!
Nought cared this body for wind or weather
When youth and I lived in't together.

Samuel Taylor Coleridge
Youth and Age

I think I am looking specially old and ugly. My youth is gone like a dream, and very little use have I ever made of it. What have I done these last thirty years? Precious little.

Charlotte Bronte
The Life of Charlotte Bronte

The older I grow, the more I distrust the familiar doctrine that age brings wisdom.

H L Mencken
Prejudices

My days are in the yellow leaf;
The flowers and fruits of love are gone;
The worm, the canker, and the grief
Are mine alone…
The hope, the fear, the jealous care,
The exalted portion of the pain
And power of love, I cannot share,
But wear the chain.

George Gordon, Lord Byron
On this Day I Complete my 36th Year

All the world's a stage,
And all the men and women merely players;
They have their exits and their entrances;
And one man in his time plays many parts
Last scene of all,
That ends this strange, eventful history,
Is second childishness and mere oblivion;
Sans teeth, sans eyes, sans taste, sans everything.

William Shakespeare
As You Like It

How can the moribund old man reason back to himself the romance, the mystery, the imminence of great things with which earth tingled for him in the days when he was young and well?

William James
The Varieties of Religious Experience

And though each morning new arise
Yet we each day grow older.

Walter Porter
Love in Thy Youth

This is not the life
I dreamt of in the garden
When I was eighteen.

Bronwen Wrigley
Summer Morning

She was experienced, adult and grown up now. But she had been happier then.

Winston Graham
Demelza

Oh how hideous it is
To see three generations of one house gathered together!
It is like an old tree with shoots,
And with some branches rotten and falling.

Ezra Pound
Commission

Deceptive images of a vague happiness hover before us in our dreams...and we search in vain for
their original.

Arthur Schopenhauer
Parerga and Paralipomena

The crumpled woman remembers when
Her feet tapped to speed up life
But now the feet are tired and old
And each step aches with dwindling hours.

Roseanne Flynn
The City People Meet Themselves

Increase of days increases misery

Branwell Bronte
The Callousness Produced by Care

Sad is our youth for it is ever going
Crumbling away beneath our very feet
Sad is our life, for onward it is flowing
In current unperceived because so fleet.
Sad are our hopes for they were rich in sowing
But tares, self-sown, have overtopped the wheat
Sad are our joys, for they were sweet in blowing
And still, Oh still, their dying breath is sweet.

Aubrey De Vere
Human Life

The child wonders at the Christmas Tree!
Let him continue to wonder
So that the glittering rapture, the amazement
Of the first remembered Christmas Tree,
So that the surprises, delight in new possessions,
(Each one with its peculiar and exciting smell)
The expectation of the goose or turkey
And the expected awe on its appearance
So that the reverence and the gaiety
May not be forgotten in later experience
In the bored habituation, the fatigue, the tedium,
The awareness of death, the consciousness of failure.

T S Eliot
The Cultivation of Christmas Trees

The older I get the more bewildering the world becomes.

Lyndon Morgans
Interview with Lyndon

When I was young – Ah, woeful when!
Ah! For the Change 'twixt now and then!

Samuel Taylor Coleridge
Youth and Age

Leaves like the things of man, you
With your fresh thoughts care for, can you?
Ah! As the heart grows older
It will come to such sights colder
By and by, nor spare a sigh
Though worlds of wanwood leafmeal lie;
And yet you will weep and know why.

Gerard Manley Hopkins
Spring and Fall

When you're young, you always feel that life hasn't yet begun – that 'life' is always scheduled to begin next week, next month, next year, after the holidays – whenever. But then suddenly you're old and the scheduled life didn't arrive.

Douglas Coupland
Life After God

Oh roses for the flush of youth,
        And laurel for the perfect prime:
But pluck an ivy branch for me
        Grown old before my time.
Oh violets for the grave of youth,
        And bay for those dead in their prime:
Give me the withered leaves I chose
        Before in the old time.

Christina Rossetti
Song

The paint's been flaking on my life for years.

Lyndon Morgans
On Porthcawl Sands

Tired of lying in the sunshine
Staying home to watch the rain;
And you are young and life is long
And there is time to kill today.
And then one day you find
Ten years have got behind you;
No one told you when to run
You missed the starting gun.
And you run, and you run to catch up with the sun,
But it's sinking,
And racing around to come up behind you again.
And the sun is the same, in a relative way
But you're older;
Shorter of breath
And one day closer to death.

Roger Waters
Time

The fundamental characteristic of old age is disillusionment; the illusions which hitherto...spurred us to activity have vanished. We have recognised the vanity and emptiness of all the splendours of the world...We have learned that there is very little behind most of the things desired and most of the pleasures hoped for; and we have gradually gained an insight into the great poverty and hollowness of our whole existence.

Arthur Schopenhauer
Essays and Aphorisms

The days of our age are three-score years and ten; and though men be so strong that they come to four-score years: yet is their strength then but labour and sorrow; so soon passeth it away, and we are gone.

Psalm 90

The briefest part of life's uncertain day,
Youth's lovely blossom, hastes to swift decay:
While love, wine, song, enhance our gayest mood
Old age creeps on, nor thought, nor understood.

Thomas Peacock
Life's Uncertain Day

Oh could I feel as I have felt, or be what I have been,
Or weep as I could once have wept...

George Gordon, Lord Byron
Youth and Age

It is autumn; not without,
    But within me is the cold.
Youth and spring are all about;
    It is I that have grown old.

Henry Wadsworth Longfellow
Autumn Within

Old age has the last word; the purely naturalistic look at life, however enthusiastically it may begin, is sure to end in sadness.

William James
The Varieties of Religious Experience

Beauty is but a flower which wrinkles will devour.

Thomas Nashe
Adieu, Farewell

That age is best which is the first
When youth and blood are warmer;
But being spent, the worse, and worst
Times still succeed the former.

Robert Herrick
Counsel to Girls

Dance there upon the shore;
What need have you to care
For wind or water's roar?
And tumble out your hair
That the salt drops have wet;
Being young, you have not known
The fool's triumph, nor yet
Love lost as soon as won,
Nor the best labourer dead
And all the sheaves to bind.
What need have you to dread
The monstrous crying of the wind?

W B Yeats
To a Child Dancing in the Wind

Alas! Regardless of their doom
    The little victims play;
No sense have they of ills to come,
    Nor care beyond today

Thomas Gray
Ode on a Distant Prospect of Eton College

Weep not, my wanton, smile upon my knee
When thou art old there's grief enough for thee.

Robert Greene
Sephesta's Song to her Child

[W]orks of art, music or poetry now... cause a whirlwind of blighting sorrow that sweeps over my mind with unspeakable dreariness...[N]early every pleasurable excitement that I used to know has changed to insipidity or pain...[At] twenty-eight I am...thoroughly old..., mentally and bodily.

Branwell Bronte
Letter to J B Leyland

Dewdrops are the gems of morning,
But the tears of mournful eve!
Where no hope is, life's a warning
That only serves to make us grieve,
When we are old!

Samuel Taylor Coleridge
Youth and Age

For some reason everyone desires to achieve old age; that is to say a condition in which one can say: "Today it is bad, and day by day it will get worse – until at last the worst of all arrives".

Arthur Schopenhauer
Essays and Aphorisms

Remember when you were young?
You shone like the sun.

Roger Waters
Shine On You Crazy Diamond

And this same flower that smiles today,
Tomorrow will be dying.

Robert Herrick
To Make Much of Time

Twenty years and the spring is over

T S Eliot
New Hampshire

Do you remember when…we were young…when we were kids, before all hope stopped?

Lyndon Morgans
Your New Best Friend

When I survey my past life, I discover nothing but a barren waste of time, with disorders of body, and disturbances of the mind very near to madness.

Samuel Johnson
Prayers and Meditations

All that age doth teach is ill.

Henry Vaughan
Childhood

Hearts are made to be broken.

Oscar Wilde
De Profundis

I gave my heart so many times. And was it worth it after all?

Will Sheff
Lady Liberty

Marriage is like life – it is a field of battle, and not a bed of roses.

Robert Louis Stevenson
Virginibus Puerisque

When love breaks down
The lies we tell,
They only serve to fool ourselves,
When love breaks down
The things you do
To stop the truth from hurting you.

Paddy McAloon
When Love Breaks Down

What do you need with fire in the blood once you get married?

Roy Clarke
Last of the Summer Wine

[T]here are many people...in marriages that show no sign of movement in any direction...Such people are often contented, not realising, perhaps, that they are going in that direction in which we all go – downwards.

Alexander McCall Smith
Espresso Tales

Love: A temporary insanity curable by marriage.

Ambrose Bierce
The Devil's Dictionary

If your arms would find me now
I know I could reveal
Oceans of pain

Emmett Tinley
I Carry This Secret

He never spoke to me. He never touched me. We stood beside one another and we were not together. We were two performers in a play, but we were divided, we were not acting with one another. We had to endure it alone; we had to put up this show, this miserable sham performance.

Daphne Du Maurier
Rebecca

So, we'll go no more a-roving
  So late into the night,
Though the heart be still as loving,
  And the moon be still as bright.

For the sword outwears its sheath,
  And the soul wears out the breast,
And the heart must pause to breathe,
  And love itself have rest.

Though the night was made for loving,
  And the day returns too soon,
Yet we'll go no more a-roving
  By the light of the moon.

George Gordon, Lord Byron
So We'll Go No More A-Roving

Every person alive has experienced the profound hurt of finding rejection when he or she has longed for acceptance. We come into marriage hoping for something different, but inevitably, we soon encounter some form of criticism or rejection. The pain that results is so intense that it demands relief. So we retreat behind protective walls of emotional distance for fear of experiencing more pain.

Larry Crabb
The Marriage Builder

Love is an incurable disease. In love, there is permanent suffering.

Marcel Proust
Unsourced

We're just two lost souls swimming in a fish bowl
Year after year. Running over the same old ground
What have we found?
The same old fears.

Roger Waters
Wish You Were Here

Don't call me or send me any more letters
I just can't stand to see your hand writing things that you don't mean.

Will Sheff
Lady Liberty

Men have a much better time of it than women. For one thing they marry later; for another they die earlier.

H L Mencken
Chrestomathy

Just when you thought you'd got used to all of life's painful surprises, along comes a Golden Wedding. [10]

Roy Clarke
Last of the Summer Wine

What of soul was left, I wonder, when the kissing had to stop?

Robert Browning
A Toccata of Galuppi's

As fast as ever Cupid shoots, the game dissolves and disappears into eternity from under his failing arrows. When the play is over we may ask what has become of these great, weighty and 'undying' loves; and they can only show us a few songs from a bygone age, a few actions worth remembering, and a few children who have retained some stamp from the disposition of their parents.

Robert Louis Stevenson
Virginibus Puerisque

Love-matches are made by people who are content, for a month of honey, to condemn themselves to a life of vinegar.

Countess of Blessington
Unsourced

Night after night we pretend it's all right
But I have grown older
And you have grown colder
And nothing is very much fun anymore.

Roger Waters
One of my Turns

Waiting for her in the usual bar
He finds she's late again.
Impatience frets at him,
But not the fearful, half-sweet pain he knew
So long ago.

That cherished perturbation is replaced
By styptic irritation
And, under that, a cold
Dark current of dejection moves
That this is so.

There was a time when all her failings were
Delights he marvelled at:
It seemed her clumsiness,
Forgetfulness and wild non-sequiturs
Could never grow.
Wearisome, nor would he ever tire
Of doting on those small
Blemishes that proved
Her beauty as the blackbird's gloss affirms
The bridal snow.

The clock above the bar records her theft
Of time he cannot spare;
Then suddenly she's here.
He stands to welcome and accuse her with
A grey "Hello".

And sees, for one slight instant, in her eyes
His own aggrieved dislike
Wince back at him before
Her smile draws blinds. "Sorry I'm late", she says.
"Where shall we go?"

Vernon Scannell
Where Shall We Go?

Broken hearted is my default mode.

Lyndon Morgans
She Lets Me in by the Back Door

My sense of adventure got lost somewhere. I remember taking it on honeymoon but coming
back without it.

Roy Clarke
Last of the Summer Wine

I waited, our faded love growing even more faded.

Will Sheff
Lady Liberty

Times are changed with him who marries; there are no more by-path meadows where you may innocently linger, but the road lies long and straight and dusty to the grave.

Robert Louis Stevenson
Virginibus Puerisque

I was never a lover. I got married instead.

Roy Clarke
The Last of the Summer Wine

One day contains the whole of my life

Samuel Johnson
The Life of Samuel Johnson

I said to my soul, be still and let the dark come upon you
Which shall be the darkness of God...
I said to my soul, be still and wait without hope
For hope would be hope for the wrong thing; there is yet
    faith
But the faith and the love and the hope are all in the waiting
Wait without thought, for you are not yet ready for thought
So the darkness shall be the light, and the stillness the dancing.

T S Eliot
Four Quartets (East Coker)

When we look carefully at what we deeply desire, we come to realise that what we want is simply not available. The more aware we become of our most passionate longings, the more lonely and sad we feel.

Larry Crabb
Inside Out

And if there was any magic I must have missed that too.

Lyndon Morgans
Gigolo Moon

Our earthly joys are almost without exception the creatures of a moment; I doubt whether any of us knows the meaning of lasting happiness. Even in our keenest pleasures there is scarcely a single moment of which the heart could truthfully say: "Would that this moment could last forever!" And how can we give the name of happiness to a fleeting state which leaves our hearts still empty and anxious, either regretting something that is past or desiring something that is yet to come?

Jean-Jacques Rousseau
Reveries of the Solitary Walker

How many of our daydreams would darken into nightmares if there seemed any danger of their coming true!

Logan Pearsall Smith
Afterthoughts (1931) 'Life and Human Nature'

The invitations by which men allure others to a state which they feel to be wretched, proceed from the natural malignity of hopeless misery. They are weary of themselves and of each other. They envy liberty and would gladly see all mankind imprisoned like themselves.

Samuel Johnson
The History of Rasselas

Is it the world, or my eyes, that are sadder?
I see not the grace that I used to see
In the meadow-brook whose song was so glad, or
In the boughs of the willow tree.
When the heart grows weary, all things seem dreary;
When the burden grows heavy, the way seems long.
Thank God for sending kind death as an ending,
Like a grand Amen to a minor song.

Ella Wheeler Wilcox
Through Dim Eyes

Unhearing unseeing you go your way. Day after day. The same way. As if there were no other any more. For you there is no other any more...Almost as if all at once the heart too heavy. In the end too heavy.

Samuel Beckett
Company

[E]verything becomes nothingness in our hands

Sigmund Freud
Civilisation and its Discontents

Oh God! If this indeed be all
That life can show to me
If on my aching brow may fall
No freshening dew from Thee.
If with no brighter sun than this
The lamp of hope may glow
And I may only dream of bliss,
And wake, to weary woe.

If life must be so full of care
Then call me soon to Thee
Or give me strength enough to bear
My load of misery.

Anne Bronte
Oh God! If This Indeed Be All

The present never satisfies us and experience deceives us and leads us on from one misfortune to another until death comes as the ultimate and eternal climax.

Blaise Pascal
Pensees

I am worn out with dreams.

W B Yeats
Men Improve with the Years

She stands staring out at the stars
Wondering at the point of it all

Lyndon Morgans
Just Another Night in Limbo

I am not sure...whether we should be so attached to existing...Do we really want to continue always to exist? Do we want to travel with our rickety identity forever?...Is there no point when we will have had *enough*?

Robert Nozick
The Examined Life

I want to be let out of this dark cavern, to open myself up to the ease of not-living. I am tired of sorrow and struggle and worry...I want to turn out the last light.

Jean Hegland
Into the Forest

The weariness of life that has no will
To climb the steepening hill:
The sickness of the soul for sleep, and to be still.

Siegfried Sassoon
Everyman

Slowly light strengthens, and the room takes shape.
It stands plain as a wardrobe, what we know,
Have always known, know that we can't escape
Yet can't accept. One side will have to go.
Meanwhile telephones crouch, getting ready to ring
In locked-up offices, and all the uncaring
Intricate rented world begins to rouse.
The sky is white as clay, with no sun.
Work has to be done.
Postmen like doctors go from house to house.

Philip Larkin
Audabe

[H]uman beings teem with desires that cannot...have any hope of being satisfied.

Joshua Foa Dienstag
Pessimism

There are times now when it appears to me as if all my ideas and feelings are changed from what they used to be. Something in me, which used to be enthusiasm, is tamed down and broken.

Charlotte Bronte
The Life of Charlotte Bronte

Through this and through no other fault we fell,
Nor, being fallen, bear other pain than this,
Always without hope in desire to dwell.

Dante
Paradise Lost

What is that corny line from that musical? *I let my golden chances pass me by.* Yes that was it;
sentimental, but absolutely true. We all let our golden chances pass us by – all the time.

Alexander McCall Smith
Espresso Tales

It's only disappointment keeps me holed up in this room,
But hell, I swam in disappointment inside my mother's womb.

Lyndon Morgans
The Time for Miracles is Past

Life is one long process of getting tired.

Samuel Butler
Note-books of Samuel Butler

[T]he more we look forward to anything, the less we enjoy it when it comes.

Arthur Schopenhauer
Studies in Pessimism

When I consider life, 'tis all a cheat,
Yet, fooled with hope, men favour the deceit;
Trust on, and think tomorrow will repay:
Tomorrow's falser than the former day;
Lies worse; and while it says we shall be blessed
With some new joys, cuts off what we possessed.
None would live past years again;
Yet all hope pleasure in what yet remain;
And from the dregs of life, think to receive,
What the first sprightly running could not give.

John Dryden
Aureng Zebe

Ah, human cares! Ah, how much futility in the world!

Lucilius
Unsourced

Very few live by choice. Every man is placed in his present condition by causes which acted without his foresight, and with which he did not always willingly co-operate; and therefore you will rarely meet one who does not think the lot of his neighbour better than his own.

Samuel Johnson
The History Of Rasselas

After each night we are emptier.

E M Cioran
A Short History of Decay

Nay, barren are those mountains and spent the streams:
Our song is the voice of desire, that haunts our dreams,
A throe of the heart,
Whose pining visions dim, forbidden hopes profound,
No dying cadence nor long sigh can sound,
For all our art.

Robert Bridges
Nightingales

There's nothing in this world can make me joy
Life is as tedious as a twice-told tale
Vexing the dull ear of a drowsy man.

William Shakespeare
King John

What is man? A wretched being
Tossed upon the tide of time
All its rocks and whirlpools seeing
Yet denied the power of fleeing
Waves and gulfs of woe and crime
Foredoomed from life's bitter breath
To launch upon the sea of death
Without hope, without a stay
To guide him on his weary way.

Branwell Bronte
What is Man?

Tomorrow we'll dream of places we'll never see.

Lyndon Morgans
In the Well of Lost Causes

If our condition were truly happy we should not need to divert ourselves from thinking about it.

Blaise Pascal
Pensees

Everyone is obsessed by what they are excluded from.

Adam Phillips
Monogamy

Art thou pale for weariness
Of climbing heaven and gazing on the earth,
Wandering companionless
Among the stars that have a different birth,
And ever changing, like a joyless eye
That finds no object worth its constancy?

P B Shelley
Art Thou Pale for Weariness?

From the bottom of every fountain of pleasure something bitter rises up and the buzz of life ceases as a piano-string stops sounding when the damper falls upon it.

William James
The Varieties of Religious Experience

[W]ho we are on the inside cannot belong in this world because we are all different, and because no one completely accepts another for their differences. Thus the plague of not belonging leaves us in search of something that cannot be found.

Ashlyn Bradley
The Plague in All of Us

Most of us spend our [lives] trying to pretend things are better than they are. When reality breaks through…we're strongly inclined to do whatever restores our feigned sense of well being. We may count our blessings, cut the lawn, pray for strength, eat something sweet…or go out with friends for a pizza – anything to get away from that nagging sense that something is missing, something is wrong. Most of us are not consciously aware of trying to get rid of personal discomfort by eating pizza. We just happen to like pizza. But more often than we know, the things we do are designed to bring relief from a vague sense of emptiness we may hardly notice.

Larry Crabb
Inside Out

The lot of man is ceaseless labour,
Or ceaseless idleness, which is still harder.

T S Eliot
Choruses From 'The Rock'

We never have a long continuation of agreeable life. It is frequently interrupted… . After every enjoyment comes weariness or disgust. We never have a large lawn of agreeable life. It is cut to pieces with sunk fences…even where it is smoothest.

James Boswell
Defence

[A]ll your tears have got you nowhere…

Emmett Tinley
In My Arms Again

Every satisfaction man attains lays the seeds of some new desire.

Arthur Schopenhauer
Studies in Pessimism

The 'normal', the 'ordinary', the 'expected' are illusions, and they are illusions which, believed in, lead to tragic consequences. People believe in romantic love, political and economic programmes, progress, dogmatic religious systems, happiness, and in many other things, including their fondest hopes; none of these work for very long.

Martin Seymour Smith
Introduction to *The Mayor of Casterbridge*

A church bell rings like it's just going through the motions, kind of like me and my life.

Lyndon Morgans
I Bought a Rose From the Guy at the Traffic Lights

If only...if only...There is an eternal longing in each of us. Why am I always so sure that the one thing I cannot attain is going to bring me happiness? This wish for an unattainable perfection is inescapable. It is the blight for which Man was born.

John Daulman
St Anne's Parish Magazine

The world is but a broken toy
Its pleasure hollow, false its joy
Unreal its loveliest hue, alas,
Its pains alone are true, alas,
Its pains alone are true.

W S Gilbert
Princess Ida

Disappointment is one of the most negative of human experiences. It is a terrible thing to see joy die in a child's eyes. It may be even worse to see the settled, dull disillusionment in the eyes of an adult who has been disappointed by life so often that he has given up hope as altogether too painful.

Maria Boulding
The Coming of God

We strew life with our blunders, our misdeeds, our lost opportunities, with all the memorials of our inadequacy.

William James
The Varieties of Religious Experience

[T]he more we strive for happiness, the further it retreats from us.

Joshua Foa Dienstag
Pessimism

Whoever you are, you may well be weary
From dragging your feet round this little star.

Paddy McAloon
Whoever You Are

All things are full of labour;...the eye is not satisfied with seeing, nor the ear filled with hearing.

Ecclesiastes 1

Inside, life still feels just as unreal as it did back in the schoolyard.

Lyndon Morgans
Interview with Lyndon

Continually it had happened that what she had desired had not been granted her, and that what had been granted her, she had not desired.

Thomas Hardy
The Mayor of Casterbridge

"What", said he, "makes the difference between man and the rest of the animal creation? Every beast that strays beside me has the same corporal necessities with myself; he is hungry and crops the grass, he is thirsty and drinks the stream and his thirst and hunger are appeased, he is satisfied and sleeps. I am hungry and thirsty like him, but when thirst and hunger cease I am not at rest; I am, like him, pained with want, but am not, like him, satisfied with fullness. The intermediate hours are tedious and gloomy. The birds fly away to the groves where they sit in seeming happiness on the branches and waste their lives in tuning one unvaried series of sounds. I likewise can call the lutanist and the singer, but the sounds that pleased me yesterday weary me today, and will grow yet more wearisome tomorrow."

Samuel Johnson
The History of Rasselas

Sleep brings no joy to me
Remembrance never dies
My soul is given to misery
And lives in sighs.

Emily Bronte
Sleep Brings No Joy

The two foes of human happiness are pain and boredom.

Arthur Schopenhauer
Essay: *Personality or What a Man Is*

We think either of present or of threatened miseries, and even if we felt quite safe on every side,
boredom would not fail to emerge from the depths of our hearts and poison our whole mind.

Blaise Pascal
Pensees

One bitter time of mourning, I remember,
When day, and night, my sad heart did complain,
My life, I said, was one cold, bleak December,
And all its pleasures, were but whited pain

Ella Wheeler Wilcox
Blind Sorrow

[S]he is dying piece-meal
of a sort of emotional anaemia...

Her boredom is exquisite and excessive.
She would like someone to speak to her,
And is almost afraid that I
will commit that indiscretion.

Ezra Pound
The Garden

We all hurt, deep down. Usually it is not a spectacular, tragic kind of hurt, but a general greyness that settles like dust over our lives – a drabness, a dullness, a dreariness, an ugliness, an ordinariness of everything. We have almost no reason to get out of bed and almost any reason to get in.

Peter Kreeft
Making Sense out of Suffering

And all my heart's voices are counting off the choices I didn't make,
All the chances I didn't take.

Lyndon Morgans
Pilgrim Hill

[I]f [the Desire] comes to a [person] while he is looking at a far off hillside he at once thinks "if only I were there"; if it comes when he is remembering some event in the past, he thinks "if only I could go back to those days"...If it comes...in a context with erotic suggestions he believes he is desiring the perfect beloved...But every one of these impressions is wrong...An easy experiment will show that by going to the far hillside you will get either nothing, or else a recurrence of the same desire which sent you thither. A...study of your own memories will prove that by returning to the past you could not find...that ecstasy which some sudden reminder of the past now moves you to desire. Those remembered moments were either quite commonplace at the time (and owe all their enchantment to memory) or else were themselves moments of desiring...As for the sexual answer, that I suppose to be the most obviously false Florimel of all. On whatever plane you take it, it is not what we are looking for. Lust can be gratified...A happy marriage can be achieved. But what has any of [these]...to do with that unnameable something, desire for which pierces us like a rapier at the smell of a bonfire, the sound of wild ducks flying overhead..., the morning cobwebs in late summer, or the noise of falling waves?

C S Lewis
The Pilgrim's Regress

I wait and what I wait for can never come.

D H Lawrence
Sons and Lovers

O, who can hold a fire in his hand
By thinking on the frosty Caucasus?
Or cloy the hungry edge of appetite
By bare imagination of a feast?
Or wallow naked in December snow
By thinking on fantastic summer's heat?
O, no! The apprehension of the good
Gives but the greater feeling to the worse:
Fell sorrow's tooth doth never rankle more
Than when it bites, but lanceth not the sore.

William Shakespeare
Richard II

Beneath the surface of everyone's life, especially the more mature, is an ache that will not go away. It can be ignored, disguised, mislabelled or submerged by a torrent of activity, but it will not disappear. And for good reason. We were designed to enjoy a better world than this. And until that better world comes along, we will groan for what we do not have. *An aching soul is evidence, not of neurosis, or spiritual immaturity, but of realism.*

Larry Crabb
Inside Out

There is not any hour complete
Nor any season satisfied!

Gerald Gould
The Search

[A]pparently diverse, our condition is instead monotonous; apparently pleasurable, our lives our instead full of...pain; apparently free, we are instead shackled.

Joshua Foa Dienstag
Pessimism

To every place of entertainment we go with expectation and desire of being pleased; we meet others who are brought by the same motives; no one will be the first to own the disappointment; one face reflects the smile of another, till each believes the rest delighted, and endeavours to catch and transmit the circulating rapture. In time, all are deceived by the cheat to which all contribute. The fiction of happiness is propagated by every tongue, and confirmed by every look, till at last all profess the joy which they do not feel.

Samuel Johnson
The Idler

Now I am here, what thou wilt do with me
None of my books will show:
I read, and sigh, and wish I were a tree –
For sure, then, I should grow
To fruit or shade; at least, some bird would trust
Her household to me, and I should be just.

George Herbert
Affliction

Our sincerest laughter
With some pain is fraught
Our sweetest songs are those that tell of saddest thought.

P B Shelley
To a Skylark

We are [always] restless, searching for the 'something else' that promises fulfilment, but ends up bringing only greater longing.

Ashlyn Bradley
The Plague in All of Us

Why do we have a need for becoming part of a fantasy world? Are our lives so sad that we envy something that does not exist?

Anon
Article: *Last of the Summer Wine*

But there are dreams that cannot be
And there are storms we cannot weather.

Herbert Kretzmer
I Dreamed a Dream

My life is what I expected it to be. Sometimes when I wake in the morning, and know that solitude, remembrance and longing are to be almost my sole companions...that at night I shall go to bed with them, that they will long keep me sleepless I have a heavy heart of it.

Charlotte Bronte
The Bronte Story

Inside I was always dead, flesh and blood was my only disguise.

Lyndon Morgans
Fairylights

The only absolute knowledge attainable by man is that life is meaningless.

Leo Tolstoy
Unsourced

How weary, stale, flat and unprofitable
Seem to me all the uses of this world.

William Shakespeare
Hamlet

Life is profoundly disappointing.

Larry Crabb
Inside Out

My heart is empty. All the fountains that should run
With longing, are in me
Dried up. In all my countryside there is not one
That drips to find the sea.
I have no care for anything thy love can grant
Except the moment's vain
And hardly noticed filling of the moment's want
And to be free from pain.

C S Lewis
The Pilgrim's Regress

[W]hile desires are perpetual, satisfactions are constantly disappearing.

Joshua Foa Dienstag
Pessimism

We give birth astride our grave. It is light for an instant and then it is night once more.

Samuel Beckett
Waiting for Godot

Tomorrow, and tomorrow, and tomorrow
Creeps in this petty pace from day to day,
To the last syllable of recorded time.

William Shakespeare
Macbeth

We…demand
Of all the thousand nothings of the hour
Their stupefying power

Matthew Arnold
The Buried Life

That old sadist time twists his knife again.

Lyndon Morgans
My Space Rock Tape

We look before and after,
And pine for what is not.

P B Shelley
To a Skylark

Time goes, you say? Ah, no! Alas, Time stays – we go.

Henry Austin Dobson
The Paradox of Time

Too much is possible
When everything is transient

Emmett Tinley
Stopping the World

Most of us cherish fond memories, which may not be very accurate, of the days when we were young…and thought that we really enjoyed life. When people…get together, they wallow in nostalgia.

Anon
Article: *The Last of the Summer Wine*

Every year is getting shorter
Never seem to find the time
Plans that either come to naught
Or half a page of scribbled lines.
Hanging on in quiet desperation is the English way
The time is gone, the song is over
Thought I'd something more to say.

Roger Waters
Time

The years go by so fast!
And one by one our loved ones pass away.
Life, health and hope today
Tomorrow comes grim death's cold bitter blast.

Colfax Burgoyne Harman
Conservatism

There was a time when meadow, grove and stream,
The earth, and every common sight,
To me did seem
Apparelled in celestial light
The glory and the freshness of a dream
It is not now as it hath been of yore;
Turn wheresoe'er I may,
By night and day,
The things which I have seen I now can see no more.

The rainbow comes and goes,
And lovely is the rose;
The moon doth with delight
Look round her when the heavens are bare;
Waters on a starry night
Are beautiful and fair;
The sunshine is a glorious birth;
But yet I know, where'er I go,
That there hath passed away a glory from the earth.

William Wordsworth
Recollections of Early Childhood

Every moment of our lives, we are on our way to death, whether we recognise this or not.

Joshua Foa Dienstag
Pessimism

Oh threats of Hell and hopes of Paradise
One thing is certain – this life flies
One thing is certain and the rest is lies;
The flower that once is blown for ever dies.

Edward Fitzgerald
Rubaiyat of Omar Khayyam

Comfort? Comfort scorn'd of devils! This is truth the poet sings,
That a sorrow's crown of sorrow is remembering happier things,
Drug thy memories, lest thou learn it, lest thy heart be put to proof,
In the dead, unhappy night, and when the rain is on the roof.

Alfred, Lord Tennyson
Locksley Hall

I have no feeling either for the future or the past, while the present seems to me poison.

E M Cioran
On the Heights of Despair

In headaches and in worry
Vaguely life leaks away,
And Time will have his fancy
Tomorrow or today.

W H Auden
As I Walked Out One Evening

You did not come,
And marching Time drew on, and wore me numb.

Thomas Hardy
A Broken Appointment

The ever-rolling silent hours
Will bring a time we shall not know
When our young days of gathering flowers
Will be an hundred years ago.

Thomas Peacock
Love and Age

This is the land of lost content
I see it shining plain
The happy highways where I went
And cannot come again.

A E Housman
A Shropshire Lad

Oh what happened to you, whatever happened to me?
What became of the people we used to be?
Tomorrow's almost over
Today went by so fast
[And] the only thing to look forward [to's]
The past.

Mike Hugg/Ian La Frenais
What Happened to You?

But your living in the past is quite different. When you do recall something that was good [or] happy, you do this with painful regret. Something, or someone, has been lost, never to return.

Dorothy Rowe
Depression

Time goes on, and the happy years are dead.

J L Molloy
The Kerry Dancing

We never keep to the present because the fact is that the present usually hurts. We thrust it out of sight because it distresses us and if we do find it enjoyable, we are sorry to see it slip away.

Blaise Pascal
Pensees

So every day we live, a day we die.

Thomas Campion
Sic Transit

All my past life is mine no more
The flying hours are gone.

John Wilmot, Earl of Rochester
Love and Life

[T]rue pleasure is evanescent and constantly receding into the past.

Joshua Foa Dienstag
Pessimism

When to the sessions of sweet silent thought
I summon up remembrance of things past,
I sigh the lack of many a thing I sought,
And with old woes new wail my dear time's waste.

William Shakespeare
Sonnet

And so we beat on, boats against the current, borne back ceaselessly into the past.

F Scott Fitzgerald
The Great Gatsby

Footfalls echo in the memory
Down the passage which we did not take
Towards the door we never opened
Into the rose garden.

T S Eliot
Four Quartets (Burnt Norton)

We have short time to stay, as you,
We have as short a spring;
As quick a growth to meet decay,
As you, or anything.
We die,
As your hours do, and dry
Away,
Like to the summer's rain;
Or as the pearls of morning's dew,
Ne'er to be found again.

Robert Herrick
To Daffodils

Time heals old pains, while it creates new ones.
Hebrew Proverb

Not the least of the torments which plague our existence is the constant pressure of time, which never lets us so much as draw breath but pursues us all like a taskmaster with a whip.

Arthur Schopenhauer
Essays and Aphorisms

Years have passed me by.

Emmett Tinley
I Carry This Secret

Tears, idle tears, I know not what they mean
Tears from the depth of some divine despair
Rise in the heart, and gather to the eyes,
In looking on the happy Autumn fields,
And thinking of the days that are no more.

Alfred, Lord Tennyson
The Princess

Memories are killing. So you must not think of certain things, of those that are dear to you, or rather you must think of them, for if you don't there is the danger of finding them, in your mind, little by little.

Samuel Beckett
The Expelled

Safe, safe – enjoy your time feeling so safe
And treasure that smile on your face
Because time will see that it's replaced

Will Sheff
Blanket and Crib

Like as the waves make towards the pebbled shore
So do our minutes hasten to their end
Each changing place with that which goes before.

William Shakespeare
Revolutions

All the tragedies which we can imagine return in the end to the one and only tragedy: the passage of time.

Simone Weil
Lectures on Philosophy

If I might see another Spring –
Oh stinging comment on my past
That all my past results in 'if'–
If I might see another Spring
I'd laugh today, today is brief;
I would not wait for anything:
I'd use today that cannot last,
Be glad today and sing.

Christina Rossetti
Another Spring

Time will say nothing but I told you so,
Time only knows the price we have to pay

W H Auden
If I Could Tell You

The irony is…that the past seems more 'real', more poignant, more acute and alive than the present…The past was wonderful because at least you were really alive then. Now you are simply alone in the dark, remembering, hardly alive at all.

Gregory Johns
In the Dim Void

Oh the happy days of doing.

W S Gilbert
Yeomen of the Guard

[T]he reality of temporal existence is transience, decay and death…

Joshua Foa Dienstag
Pessimism

"I just feel that my past is getting larger, my future's getting smaller and I haven't got time for the present", said Bob, one of the heroes of the TV series, 'Whatever Happened to the Likely Lads?'...Bob's words, uttered in his usual rueful, anxious way, made us laugh – the kind of laugh that comes when we are presented with something which we know is, sadly, only too true about ourselves.

Dorothy Rowe
Depression

So when the close of pleasure's day
To gloom has near consigned us
We turn to catch one fading ray
Of joy that's left behind us.

Thomas Moore
The Journey Onwards

Time hovers o'er, impatient to destroy,
And shuts up all the passages of joy.

Samuel Johnson
The Vanity of Human Wishes

One day when God says He can no longer stand to bear witness
And He's saving the last round in the chamber for Himself
I'll be parked on some slip road, drunk and nostalgic
For the roads I took, when I still cared where I was going.

Lyndon Morgans
One Day When God Begs My Forgiveness

Time is our enemy not easily slain.

Emmett Tinley
Millionaire Hero

The future is a faded song, a lavender spray
Of wistful regret
Pressed between yellow leaves of a book that has never been
opened
You cannot face it steadily, but this thing is sure,
That time is no healer

T S Eliot
Four Quartets (The Dry Salvages)

There is no escape from yesterday because yesterday has deformed us or been deformed by us.

Samuel Beckett
Proust

Time does not bring relief; you all have lied
Who told me time would ease me of my pain!

Edna St Vincent Millay
Time Does Not Bring Relief

He seems
To have seen better days, as who has not
Who has seen yesterday?

George Gordon, Lord Byron
Werner

There is no greater sorrow than thinking back upon a happy time in misery

Dante
Inferno

But were there any
Writhed not at passed joy?
To know the change and feel it
When there is none to heal it?

John Keats
Happy Insensibility

She cries herself to sleep to drown the sound of time unravelling.

Lyndon Morgans
The Way of the World

We mortal millions live alone.

Matthew Arnold
To Marguerite Continued

Jealousy is no more than feeling alone against smiling enemies.

Elizabeth Bowen
The House in Paris

The family is the source of our deepest hurts. If you are part of a family, you know how those closest to you hurt you the most.

Peter Kreeft
Making Sense out of Suffering

The mind blanks at the glare. Not in remorse
The good not used, the love not given, time
Torn off unused – nor wretchedly because
An only life can take so long to climb
Clear of its wrong beginnings, and may never:
But at the total emptiness forever,
The sure extinction that we travel to
And shall be lost in always. Not to be here,
Not to be anywhere,
And soon; nothing more terrible, nothing more true.

Philip Larkin
Audabe

Loneliness is…the central and inevitable fact of human existence.

Thomas Wolfe
Unsourced

There has to be someone to hold you
Every day, someone to need you
To make a fire out of the grey confusion.

Emmett Tinley
Polichinelle

And you as you always were. Alone.

Samuel Beckett
Company

There was a door
And I could not open it, I could not touch the handle
Why could I not walk out of my prison?
What is Hell? Hell is oneself
Hell is alone, the other figures in it merely projections.
There is nothing to escape from
And nothing to escape to.
Hell is always alone.

T S Eliot
The Cocktail Party

And it felt good, I didn't feel like me at all...

Lyndon Morgans
A Wretched Sinner's Song

Are we not all flung into the world only to hate each other, and therefore to torment ourselves and others?

Leo Tolstoy
Anna Karenina

The tragedy of it is that nobody sees the look of desperation on my face. Thousands and thousands of us, and we're passing one another without a look of recognition.

Henry Miller
Black Spring

In this city, perhaps a street.
In this street, perhaps a house.
In this house, perhaps a room
And in this room a woman sitting,
Sitting in the darkness, sitting and crying
For someone who had just gone through the door
Who has just switched off the light
Forgetting she was there.

Alan Brownjohn
In this City

We're all of us sentenced to solitary confinement inside our own skins, for life!

Tennessee Williams
Orpheus Descending

Yet winter comes
And you're frozen, alone,
The cornfield harvested,
The poppies gone.
And nothing is ever
Quite like it seems
So how can I live
Like I do in my dreams?

Charlotte A Wrigley
The Vagabond

We are all vulnerable and afraid...in our different ways.

Alexander McCall Smith
44 Scotland Street

I don't need no arms around me
I don't need no drug to calm me
I have seen the writing on the wall
Don't think I need anything at all
All in all it was all just bricks in the wall
All in all you were all just bricks in the wall.

Roger Waters
Another Brick in the Wall

Unrhymed, unrhythmical, the chatter goes:
Yet no one hears his own remarks as prose.
Beneath each topic tunelessly discussed
The ground-bass is reciprocal mistrust.

The names in fashion shuttling to and fro
Yield, when deciphered, messages of woe.
You cannot read me like an open book.
I'm more myself than you will ever look.

Will no one listen to my little song?
Perhaps I shan't be with you very long.
A howl for recognition, shrill with fear,
Shakes the jam-packed apartment, but each ear
Is listening to its hearing, so none hear.

W H Auden
At the Party

You've been used, you've been betrayed.

Will Sheff
Lady Liberty

When I find where I'm standing, I'm alone – always.

Emmett Tinley
Soon the Stars Will Steer Me

The lights are extinguished...
with a movement of darkness on darkness,
And the conversation rises and slowly fades into silence
And you see behind every face the mental emptiness deepen
Leaving only the growing terror of nothing to think about.

T S Eliot
Four Quartets (East Coker)

You will never be anything but what you are not, and the despair of being what you are.

E M Cioran
A Short History of Decay

And long we try in vain to speak and act
Our hidden self, and what we say and do
Is eloquent, is well – but 'tis not true!

Matthew Arnold
The Buried Life

Calamities are of two kinds: misfortune to ourselves, and good fortune to others.

Ambrose Bierce
The Devil's Dictionary

I will be dying inside
When you bring me your bunch
Of garage flowers.

Bronwen Wrigley
Unwanted Gift

[Y]ou are filled with bitterness and jealousy. Bitter that your life has gone awry and jealous that other people...do not suffer as you do. You hate yourself for feeling such...jealousy and for being unable to love...Irritable and miserable, you push others away from you, and then get scared that they will go [away[and leave you alone. So you pretend everything is all right. You try [to] smile and be ordinary, but the pretence is so wearying, and inside you are silently screaming.

Dorothy Rowe
Depression

God strengthen me to bear myself;
That heaviest weight of all to bear,
Inalienable weight of care.
All others are outside myself;
I lock my door and bar them out,
The turmoil, tedium, gad about.
I lock my door upon myself,
And bar them out; but who shall wall
Self from myself, most loathed of all?

God harden me against myself,
This coward with pathetic voice
Who craves for ease and rest and joys

Myself, arch traitor to myself;
My hollowest friend, my deadliest foe,
My clog whatever road I go.

Christina Rossetti
Who Shall Deliver Me?

Far too late in the game
You'll find that you have been betrayed,
Propped up and pushed into your place.
I could claim that it all would go great,
But the reason I came is to say that it won't.

Will Sheff
Blanket and Crib

" What do you do from morning to night?". "I endure myself."

E M Cioran
The Trouble With Being Born

Nobody heard him, the dead man,
But still he lay moaning:
I was much further out than you thought
And not waving but drowning.

Poor chap, he always loved larking
And now he's dead.
It must have been too cold for him, his heart gave way
They said.

Oh no no no, it was too cold always
(Still the dead one lay moaning):
I was much too far out all my life
And not waving but drowning.

Stevie Smith
Not Waving but Drowning

Whatever side I take, I know that I will be blamed.

King Louis XIV
Unsourced

We wait. We are bored..., bored to death...A diversion comes along and what do we do? We let it go to waste...In an instant all will vanish and we'll be alone once more in the midst of nothingness!

Samuel Beckett
Waiting for Godot

She was homesick, perpetually trembling and uneasy, haunted by morbid fancies and hysterical with loneliness and depression.

Margaret Lane
The Bronte Story

I don't feel so strong
I speak and it all goes wrong.

Emmett Tinley
Dead Flowers

I am feeble, and sore smitten: I have roared for the very disquietness of my heart.
Lord, thou knowest all my desire: and my groaning is not hid from thee.
My heart panteth, my strength hath failed me: and the sight of mine eyes is gone from me.
My neighbours did stand looking upon my trouble: and my kinsmen stood afar off.
I have required that they should not triumph over me: for when my foot slipped, they rejoiced greatly against me.
And I, truly, am set in the plague: and my heaviness is ever in my sight.

Psalm 38

Everybody out there is hurting. And if you don't know that, you're either very naive and believe people's facades, or so thick-skinned that you don't hurt yourself and don't feel other people's hurts either.

Peter Kreeft
Making Sense out of Suffering

The more I see of the world, the more am I dissatisfied with it; and every day confirms my belief
of the inconsistency of all human characters...

Jane Austen
Pride and Prejudice

She was alone, but she was used to it. The world seemed a dreary place, where nothing else would happen for her. Nothing but this dreary endurance. And looking ahead, the prospect of her life made her feel as if she were buried alive.

D H Lawrence
Sons and Lovers

How little any of us know of the real internal state even of those who we see most frequently.

James Boswell
The Life of Samuel Johnson

I weep much in my loneliness;
Autumn has lasted too long in my heart.
Sun of love, will you never shine again,
And gently dry my bitter tears?

Gustav Mahler
Das Lied

We are alone. We cannot know, and we cannot be known.

Samuel Beckett
Proust

Am I the only one who feels a nagging sense that something is badly twisted within me?

Larry Crabb
Inside Out

We are so lonely in life.

E M Cioran
On the Heights of Despair

Everywhere is emptiness
And everyone is loneliness

Emmett Tinley
Polichinelle

I should really like to think there's something wrong with me
Because, if there isn't, then there's something wrong

T S Eliot
The Cocktail Party

I wish you could stand inside and see all my bad days
Now I stand all alone at the foot of the stairs
And I wait for more bad days.

Will Sheff
My Bad Days

[We] look for love in every way that we can. We play [football] so our father will give us his nod of approval. We dress to impress in order that people will look our way and make us feel valued by their noticing us. We indulge in…sex, alcohol and drugs to delude ourselves into feeling that we are loved and accepted. We get married hoping that the love we find there will be enough to fulfil our longing. Still…we hear the piercing call for unconditional love that has not been met. And so, we are plagued…deep down, day after day, by the feeling of being unloved.

Ashlyn Bradley
The Plague in All of Us

But hardly have we, for one little hour…
Been ourselves
Hardly had skill to utter one of all
The nameless feelings that course through our breast
But they course on for ever unexpressed.

Matthew Arnold
The Buried Life

Descend lower, descend only
Into the world of perpetual solitude…
Internal darkness, deprivation
And destitution

T S Eliot
Four Quartets (Burnt Norton)

She was…totally unused to have her pleasure consulted, or to have anything take place at all in the way she could desire.

Jane Austen
Mansfield Park

Man would fain be great and sees that he is little; would fain be happy and sees that he is miserable; would fain be perfect and sees that he is full of imperfections; would fain be the object of the love and esteem of men, and sees that his faults merit only their aversion and contempt.

Blaise Pascal
Pensees

A door just opened on a street –
I, lost, was passing by –
An instant's width of warmth disclosed
And wealth, and company.
The door as sudden shut, and I,
I, lost, was passing by, –
Lost doubly, but by contrast most,
Enlightening misery.

Emily Dickinson
A Door Just Opened

[H]e...sat and reflected on loneliness and on how few, how very few, are the human bonds that lie between us and the state of being completely alone.

Alexander McCall Smith
Espresso Tales

We're all of us ill in one way or another.

T S Eliot
The Family Reunion

I am absolutely persuaded that I am nothing in this universe

E M Cioran
On the Heights of Despair

We wish we were better than we are, but we're not. And that realisation brings shame, a desire to hide, to avoid real contact, to present to others only that part of us we think will be well received...We live for the purpose of self-protection, clinging to whatever brings us...security. The effect is a discouraging distance between [ourselves] and the people we long to be close to.

Larry Crabb
Inside Out

In every face I meet
Marks of weakness, marks of woe.

William Blake
London

Could you not watch with me
Tonight, on this, the final
Evening of my life?

Bronwen Wrigley
Gethsemane

I...cannot...be flatter or older in mind than I am now.

Anne Bronte
Anne Bronte's Diary Paper

All things to end are made.

Thomas Nashe
Adieu, Farewell

This thought is as death, which cannot choose
But weep to have that which it fears to lose.

William Shakespeare
Time and Love

Ships that pass in the night, and speak each other in passing,
Only a signal shown, and a distant voice in the darkness;
So on the ocean of life, we pass and speak one another,
Only a look and a voice, then darkness again and a silence.

Henry Wadsworth Longfellow
Tales of a Wayside Inn

Everything may soon be over.

Emmett Tinley
Dark Green

'Tis a sight to engage me, if anything can,
To muse on the perishing pleasures of man;
Though his life be a dream, his enjoyments, I see,
Have a being less durable even than he.

William Cowper
The Poplar Field

I've lost everything!

E M Cioran
On the Heights of Despair

All, all are gone
The old familiar faces.

Charles Lamb
The Old Familiar Faces

I know that all beneath the moon decays
And what by mortals in this world is brought,
In time's great periods shall return to nought;
That fairest states have fatal nights and days.

William Drummond
I Know That All Beneath the Moon Decays

The central trauma of human life is separation…Every newborn human comes face to face with his first object, his mother, only to begin gradually to lose her. This primal catastrophe is the harbinger of all the losses and separations that await us all in human life, and indeed is paradigmatic of all of life's later suffering.

J L McNish
Cross Currents

Ah fading joy, how quickly art thou past!
Yet we thy ruin haste.
As if the cares of human life were few,
We seek out new:
And follow fate, which would too fast pursue.

John Dryden
The Indian Emperor

Everything just fizzles out

Lyndon Morgans
On Porthcawl Sands

All paradises are lost paradises.

Marcel Proust
In Search of Lost Time

Did not he all create
To die again? All ends that was begun
Their times in his eternal book of fate
Are written sure, and have their certain date.

Edmund Spenser
The Faerie Queene

But what of life whose bitter hungry sea
Flows at our heels, and gloom of sunless night
Covers the days which never more return?
Ambition, love and all the thoughts that burn
We lose too soon, and only find delight
In withered husks of some dead memory.

Oscar Wilde
Despair

There is a feeling that everything must end – the music, ourselves, the moon, everything. That if you get to the heart of things, you find sadness for ever and ever, everywhere.

John Fowles
The Collector

Let us alone. Time driveth onward fast,
And in a little while our lips are dumb.
Let us alone. What is it that will last?
All things are taken from us, and become
Portions and parcels of the dreadful past.

Alfred, Lord Tennyson
The Lotus-Eaters

Farewell, all joys; O death, come close mine eyes;
More geese than swans now live, more fools than wise.

Orlando Gibbons
The Silver Swan

Life gets you in the end.

Roy Clarke
Last of the Summer Wine

[It] was over; even though she rebelled against the fact she knew that it was so. She felt faint and sick, and desperately tired of being alive…[But] [t]here were no tears in her. The wound went too deep…Hers would be the perpetual ache of loss and loneliness, slowly dulled with time until it became a part of her character, a faint sourness tinged with withered pride…

[And] this room which had seen her grow to maturity would see her dry up and fade… All these ornaments and furnishings would be her companions through the years to come. And she realised that she would come to hate them…, as one hates the witnesses of one's humiliation and futility.

Winston Graham
Ross Poldark

Did you know it was all going to go so wrong for you?…
[D]id you ever realise what you'd become?
And did you know…that you'd lose that light in your eyes?

David Gilmour
Poles Apart

The pine-scented wood,
The cool of the Scottish glen
Are lost to me now.

Bronwen Wrigley
Lost World

I heard the old men say
"Everything alters
And one by one we drop away
All that's beautiful drifts away
Like the waters".

W B Yeats
The Old Men Admiring Themselves

You can grieve over the loss of more than just people. What about grieving over the loss of childhood, and so fearing to grow up? What about grieving over the loss of youth [and] beauty… and so seeing yourself [as] no longer desirable while dreaded old age approaches? Or are you mourning a dream, something that was once bright and lovely, but now unrealisable in this hard, cruel world? There will be no promised land, no happy ending. Such losses are hard to name, and even harder to mourn.

Dorothy Rowe
Depression

Change and decay in all around I see.

Henry Lyte
Abide With Me

[T]he greater part of our life is wilting away…

Giacomo Leopardi
The Moral Essays

Life death does end and each day dies with sleep.

Gerard Manley Hopkins
No Worst, There is None

Out of the day and night
A joy has taken flight;
Fresh spring, and summer, and winter hoar,
Move my faint heart with grief, but with delight
No more – oh, never more

P B Shelley
A Lament

There's not a joy the world can give like that it takes away
When the glow of early thought declines in feeling's dull decay

George Gordon, Lord Byron
Youth and Age

I cannot tell you what it was;
But this I know: it did but pass.
It passed away with sunny May,
With all sweet things it passed away,
And left me old, and cold, and grey.

Christina Rossetti
May

We lost the dreams that we once had
How did our lives turn out so bad?

Richard Hawley
Lady's Bridge

The tender grace of a day that is dead
Will never come back to me.

Alfred, Lord Tennyson
Ulysses

All natural goods perish. Riches take wings; fame is a breath; love is a cheat; youth and health and pleasure vanish.

William James
The Varieties of Religious Experience

Nothing lasts for ever
Inside every one of us there's only so long.

Ricky Ross
I Was Right

You look at the full green trees on a warm summer's day, or else at the waves beating under the cliff; and the power of the experience is an amalgamation of joy and woe. You want to be able to capture the scene and preserve it. But you cannot.

Peter Mullen
Death be not Proud

But the best I've known
Stays here, and changes, breaks, grows old, is blown
About the winds of the world, and fades from brains
Of living men, and dies.
Nothing remains.

Rupert Brooke
The Great Lover

Do you remember when we thought we had forever
Didn't it make you feel secure?
We used to think that we had forever
But now we're not so sure.

Mike Hugg/Ian la Frenais
Remember When?

Are you ready to believe it's true
That everything we love we lose?

Emmett Tinley
Polichinelle

She only knew the birth and death
Of days, when each that died
Was still at morn a hope, at night
A hope unsatisfied.

The dark trees shivered to behold
Another day begin
She, being hopeless, did not weep
As the grey dawn came in.

Arthur Symons
At Dawn

There are no permanent things; only fleeting moments of warmth and companionship, precious stationary seconds in a flicker of troubled days.

Winston Graham
Jeremy Poldark

Even such is time, which takes in trust
Our youth, our joys and all we have,
And pays us but with age and dust;
Who, in the dark and silent grave,
When we have wandered all our ways
Shuts up the story of our days.

Walter Raleigh
The Author's Epitaph

They are not long, the days of wine and roses.

Ernest Dowson
Envoy

Bid us sigh on from day to day,
And wish and wish the soul away,
Till youth and genial years are flown,
And all the life of life is gone.

Samuel Beckett
Watt

People change and smile; but the agony abides.

T S Eliot
Four Quartets (The Dry Salvages)

Why did I not perish at birth,
and die as I came from the womb?
For now I would be lying down in peace; I would be asleep and at rest.

Book of Job

Life is just a long, drawn out agony.

E M Cioran
On the Heights of Despair

Peace, peace! He is not dead, he doth not sleep –
He hath awakened from the dream of life –
'Tis we, who lost in stormy visions, keep
With phantoms an unprofitable strife,
And in mad trance, strike with our spirit's knife
Invulnerable nothings…
He has outsoared the shadow of our night;
Envy and calumny and hate and pain,
And that unrest which men miscall delight;
Can touch him not and torture not again;
From the contagion of the world's slow stain
He is secure, and now can never mourn
A heart grown cold, a head grown grey in vain…

P B Shelley
Adonais

If we see a light at the end of the tunnel, it's the light of an oncoming train.

Robert Lowell
Day by Day

The thought of suicide is a great consolation: by means of it one gets successfully through many a bad night.

Friedrich Nietzsche
Beyond Good and Evil

The sickened heart, the blasting sorrow,
The ghastly night, the ghastlier morrow,
The aching sense of utter woe

The burning tears that would keep welling,
The groans that mocked at every tear.

Emily Bronte
The Dream of Horror

We all live in a house on fire, no fire department to call; no way out, just the upstairs window to look out of while the fire burns the house down with us trapped, locked in it.

Tennessee Williams
The Milk Train Doesn't Stop Here Anymore

Do you know what it is to live among the tombs, when life seems to go dead and what once caused you pleasure and delight now leaves you unmoved, so that you live in a state of listlessness and apathy? Do you understand what it means 'to howl and gash yourself' with bitterness and resentment at what others have done to you or what you have done to yourself?

Gerard Hughes
God of Surprises

Draw on, sweet Night, best friend unto those cares
That do arise from painful melancholy.
My life so ill through want of comfort fares,
That unto thee I consecrate it wholly.
Sweet Night, draw on! My griefs when they be told
To shades and darkness, find some ease from paining
And while thou all in silence dost enfold,
I then shall have best time for my complaining.

Anon
Draw on Sweet Night

The normal process of life contains moments as bad as any of those which insane melancholy is filled with. Our civilisation is founded on the shambles, and every individual existence goes out in a lonely spasm of helpless agony. If you protest, my friend, wait till you arrive there yourself!

William James
The Varieties of Religious Experience

All the world is dying. It is just a matter of time. Time is a death factor, not a life factor. We charge a battery, it runs down. We recharge it, or couple another one on to the circuit, but ultimately, all the batteries will run down. So we die. And our dying today is an average three score years and ten of frustration and pain.

Really we are in general very brave people to struggle on. Some, not so brave, give up the struggle. Or maybe they have a form of bravery. Most of us would 'rather bear the ills we have than fly to others that we know not of'. So we push away the idea in activities.

G L Hulme
The Return of Man

[T]his world is all rottenness

Branwell Bronte
Letter to J H Thompson

Some days it feels like I'm falling apart,
Like I'm God's broken heart

Lyndon Morgans
Jinetera

To think…is to be full of sorrow
And leaden-eyed despairs.

John Keats
Ode to a Nightingale

Your disabilities are more obvious expressions of our common pain. I can see your limp, but you don't recognise the paralysis within me. T S Eliot said that we all, to a greater or lesser extent, prepare a face to meet the other faces we meet. As a philosopher said, "Most men live lives of quiet desperation".

John Daulman
St. Anne's Parish Magazine

"Month after month", he cried, "to bear this load
And as a jade urged by the whip and goad
To drag life on, which like a heavy chain
Lengthens behind with many a link of pain! –
And not to speak my grief – O not to dare
To give a human voice to my despair
But live and move, and wretched thing! smile on
As if I never went aside to groan."

P B Shelley
Julian and Maddalo: A Conversation

[M]an's condition is tragic.

E M Cioran
On the Heights of Despair

We all know at times what it is like to be wearied in spirits. Mine, I confess, are exhausted.

Jane Austen
Emma

I dreamed a dream in time gone by
When hope was high and life worth living
I dreamed that love would never die
I dreamed that God would be forgiving.

When I was young and unafraid
And dreams were made and used and wasted
There was no ransom to be paid
No song unsung, no wine untasted.

I had a dream my life would be
So different from this hell I'm living
So different now from what it seemed
Now life has killed the dream I dreamed.

Herbert Kretzmer
I Dreamed a Dream

I condemn that nature which, with such impudent nerve, brought me into being in order to suffer.

Fyodor Dostoyevsky
Diary of a Writer

One thing and only one is left me, the wish that I had never existed.

William Cowper
Letter to Cousin

Sleep is good, Death is better, yet
Surely the best thing would be to have never been born at all.

Heinrich Heine
Death and His Brother Sleep (Morphine)

Most of our hopes are bound to be disappointed.

Joshua Foa Dienstag
Pessimism

At first thou gavest me milk and sweetnesses;
I had my wish and way:
My days were strewed with flowers and happiness:
There was no month but May.
But with my years sorrow did twist and grow,
And made a party unawares of woe.
My flesh began unto my soul in pain,
Sicknesses cleave my bones,
Consuming agues dwell in every vein,
And tune my breath to groans,
Sorrow was all my soul; I scarce believed,
Till grief did tell me roundly, that I lived.

George Herbert
Affliction

My courage, my spirit – it's so much less than it was.

Richard Adams
Watership Down

The ‘morbid melancholy’ which was lurking in Johnson’s constitution and that aversion to regular life which marked his character, gathered such strength as to affect him in a dreadful manner. He felt himself overwhelmed with a horrible hypochondria, with perpetual irritation, fretfulness and impatience, and with a dejection, gloom and despair which made existence misery. From this dismal malady he never was perfectly relieved; and all his labours, and enjoyments were but temporary interruptions of its baleful influence.

James Boswell
The Life of Samuel Johnson

I’m too tired to smile

Will Sheff
The Velocity Of Saul at the Time of His Conversion

I cannot contribute anything to this world because I have only one method: agony.

E M Cioran
On the Heights of Despair

If only my anguish could be weighed
and all my misery be placed on the scales!
It would surely outweigh the sand of the seas

Book of Job

Tired with all these, for restful death I cry.

William Shakespeare
Sonnet

I have experienced
The worst the world can wreak on me – the worst
That can make life indifferent...
I have beheld the whole of all, wherein
My heart had any interest in this life,
To be disrent and torn from off my hopes
That nothing now is left. Why then live on?

Samuel Taylor Coleridge
Despair

Living is an illness to which sleep provides relief every sixteen hours. But it's just a palliative. The remedy is death.

Nicolas-Sebastien Chamfort
Maximes Et Pensees

The worst of it is that there is no way back...We have lost not only the perfect, but also our ability to earn, perform or retrieve the perfect. We truly live in *Paradise Lost.* There's no way back.

But we have not lost our *memory* of Paradise or our *need* or *desire* for it. God left the longing for the perfect within us. This longing is one of the basic hungers which characterises humans – like the hunger for...security, belongingness, affirmation, affection...and, above all, the need to love and be loved... . This gnawing nostalgia for perfection is an integral part of the...blank within us.

David Seamands
Healing Grace

Amid the sufferings of life on earth, suicide is God's best gift to man.

Pliny the Elder
Natural History

Yet now despair itself is mild,
Even as the winds and waters are;
I could lie down like a tired child
And weep away the life of care
Which I have borne and yet must bear, –
Till Death like Sleep might steal on me

P B Shelley
Stanzas Written in Dejection Near Naples

Living's just as hard as dying.

Lyndon Morgans
She Hangs in the Dark Like a Saint in a Cathedral

I wake and feel the fell of dark, not day.
What hours, O what black hours we have spent
This night! What sights you, heart, saw; ways you went!
And more must, in yet longer light's delay.

Gerard Manley Hopkins
I Wake and Feel the Fell of Dark

Only the truly stupid are happy. It means they don't know what's going on.

Suzy
My Miserable Life

Nothing perceived
Is really as it is
The world is a lie
More beautiful than herself.

Emmett Tinley
Stopping the World

Save me, O God: for the waters are come in, even unto my soul. I stick fast in the deep mire, where no ground is: I am come into deep waters, so that the floods run over me.
I am weary of crying; my throat is dry: my sight faileth me

Psalm 69

[C]onflicting instincts exist in all of us. We know that we are going to die; we do not really believe it. We want to be happy and to give happiness; [but] we know that...we shall be frustrated, and in trying to make others happy, more often than not will fail, and we know that others will fail to make us happy, too.

Rachel Trickett
No Alternative

Forever be accursed the star under which I was born.

E M Cioran
A Short History of Decay

Work, worry, toil and trouble are the lot of almost all men their whole life long.

Arthur Schopenhauer
Essays and Aphorisms

So go on, smile that's your style,
And no one would call it denial
For you're not even sure what's in store.
But it's more than you'll be able to take standing up straight.
And it won't be okay

Will Sheff
Blanket and Crib

Happiness in intelligent people is the rarest thing I know.

Ernest Hemingway
The Garden of Eden

Even if we suppose a man so packed with healthy-mindedness as never to have experienced in his own person any sobering intervals, still, if he is a reflecting being, he must generalise and class his own lot with that of others; and, doing so, he must see that his escape is just a lucky chance. He might just as well have been born to an entirely different fortune. And then indeed the hollow security! What kind of a frame of things is it of which the best you can say is, "Thank God, it has let me off clear this time!".

William James
The Varieties of Religious Experience

Why is light given to those in misery
And life to the bitter of soul?
To those who long for death that does not come
Who search for it more than hidden treasure?

Book of Job

Disease, betrayal, bereftness, suffering, death...these are first of all experiences which happen to human beings...The psalmist speaks of 'going heavily', 'the valley of the shadow' and the God who has absented himself. Beckett writes about boredom and worry, tedium and the sense of being oppressed by nothingness. These are different expressions of a recognisably similar experience...And one thing...is clear, and ought to be so even to the most glib religious enthusiast: no one who has not visited those depths and felt the barrenness and forsakeness which reside near the centre of human experience should be allowed to speak to us of God.

Peter Mullen
The New Babel

You dozed, and watched the night revealing
The thousand sordid images
Of which your soul was constituted

T S Eliot
Preludes

I talked to him of misery being "the doom of man", in this life…Yet I observed that things were done upon the supposition of happiness; grand houses were built, fine gardens were made, splendid places of public amusement were contrived, and crowded with company. Johnson: "Alas, Sir, these are all only struggles for happiness…and the thoughts of each individual there, would be distressing when alone." This reflection was experimentally just…for when the mind is vacant, a thousand disappointments and vexations rush in and excruciate.

James Boswell
The Life of Samuel Johnson

I wonder if anyone is ever truly happy?

Jack Russell
Poldark (TV Series)

Everybody knows that life isn't worth living. And when it comes down to it…it doesn't matter very much whether you die at thirty or at seventy.

Albert Camus
The Outsider

Messing up must just be written in my DNA

Lyndon Morgans
Just Another Night in Limbo

What say you now? What comfort have I now?
By heaven, I'll hate him everlastingly
That bids me be of comfort any more
        let no man speak again
To alter this, for counsel is but vain
        He does me double wrong
That wounds me with the flatteries of his tongue.

William Shakespeare
Richard II

Waking, another form of weariness awaits us; after having had just time enough to forget the night's, we are at grips with the dawn's.

E M Cioran
A Short History of Decay

[O]rdinary human life is so full of misery that it is perfectly sensible...to consider giving it up.

Joshua Foa Dienstag
Pessimism

You must go by the way wherein there is no ecstasy.

T S Eliot
Four Quartets (East Coker)

She had learnt the lesson of renunciation and was as familiar with the wreck of each day's wishes as with the diurnal setting of the sun.

Thomas Hardy
The Mayor of Casterbridge

Who will give me tears? Come, all ye springs,
Dwell in my head and eyes; come, clouds and rain;
My grief hath need of all the watery things
That nature hath produced: let every vein
Suck up a river to supply mine eyes,
My weary weeping eyes, too dry for me,
Unless they get new conduits, new supplies,
To bear them out, and with my state agree.
What are two shallow fords, two little spouts
Of a less world? The greater is but small,
A narrow cupboard for my griefs and doubts,
Which want provision in the midst of all.
Verses, ye are too fine a thing, too wise
For my rough sorrows; cease, be dumb and mute,
Give up your feet and running to mine eyes,
And keep your measures for some lover's lute,
Whose grief allows him music and a rhyme;
For mine excludes both measure, tune, and time

George Herbert
Grief

Every man may, by examining his own mind, guess what passes in the minds of others: when you feel that your own gaiety is counterfeit, it may justly lead you to suspect that of your companions not to be sincere. Envy is commonly reciprocal. We are long before we are convinced that happiness is never to be found, and each believes it possessed by others, to keep alive the hope of obtaining it for himself.

Samuel Johnson
The History of Rasselas

Life as we find it is too hard for us; it entails too much pain, too many disappointments, impossible tasks. We cannot do without palliative remedies...powerful diversions of interest which lead us to care little about our misery; substitutive gratifications, which lessen it; and intoxicating substances which make us insensitive to it.

Sigmund Freud
Civilisation and its Discontents

I looked for that which is not, nor can be,
And hope deferred made my heart sick in truth:
But years must pass before a hope of youth
Is resigned utterly.

I watched and waited with a steadfast will:
And though the object seemed to flee away
That I so longed for, ever day by day
I watched and waited still.

Sometimes I said: "This thing shall be no more;
My expectation wearies and shall cease;
I will resign it now and be at peace":
Yet never gave it o'er.
Sometimes I said: "It is an empty name
I long for; to a name why should I give
The peace of all the days I have to live?" –
Yet gave it all the same.
Alas, thou foolish one! Alike unfit
For healthy joy and salutary pain:
Thou knowest the chase useless, and again
Turnest to follow it.

Christina Rossetti
A Pause for Thought

How can things so insecure as the successful experiences of this world afford a stable anchorage? A chain is no stronger than its weakest link, and life is a chain. In the healthiest and most prosperous existence, how many links of illness, danger, and disaster are always interposed?

William James
The Varieties of Religious Experience

We're all of us resigned to death: it's life we aren't resigned to.

Graham Greene
The Heart of the Matter

I used to think life
Meant walking barefoot on a
Cornish beach. It doesn't.

Bronwen Wrigley
Reality

Happy New Year I guess (due allowance being made for that sorrow found deep down at the heart of all things, of course).

Lyndon Morgans
Lyndon's Diary

All of us are miserable, but how many know it?

E M Cioran
A Short History of Decay

Some terrible things happen behind those rose-covered cottage doors.

John Daulman
Private Conversation

The life of woman is full of woe,
Toiling on and on and on,
With breaking heart, and tearful eyes,
The secret longings that arise,
Which this world never satisfies!
Some more, some less, but of the whole
Not one quite happy, no, not one!

Henry Wadsworth Longfellow
Christus

States of human happiness can as a rule be compared with groups of trees: seen from a distance they look beautiful, but if you go up to them, their beauty disappears and you can no longer discover it. That is why we so often feel envy for other people.

Arthur Schopenhauer
Essays and Aphorisms

To drudge in furrows till you drop
Is to be born.

George Mackay Brown
First Fall

I am silent because I have literally nothing to say. My life is a pale blank, a very weary burden. The future appals me.

Charlotte Bronte
The Life of Charlotte Bronte

Enlarge my life with multitude of days!
In health, in sickness, thus the suppliant prays;
Hides from himself his state and shuns to know,
That life protracted is protracted woe.

Samuel Johnson
The Vanity of Human Wishes

My heart aches, and a drowsy numbness pains
My sense, as though of hemlock I had drunk.

John Keats
Ode to a Nightingale

Crying is common in this world. Laughter can be heard here and there, but by and large, weeping predominates. With maturity the reason for crying changes, but never does it stop. All infants do it everywhere – even in public. By adulthood most crying is done alone and in the dark. Weeping, for babies, is a sign of health and evidence that they are alive. Isn't this a chilling omen? Not laughter but tears is the sign of life.

Calvin Miller
The Valiant Papers

Let us then resolutely turn our backs on the sky-blue optimistic gospel; let us not simply cry out, in spite of all appearances, "Hurrah for the Universe! – God's in his Heaven, all's right with the world." Let us see rather whether pity, pain, and fear, and the sentiment of human helplessness may not open a profounder view.

William James
Varieties of Religious Experience

Human kind cannot bear very much reality.

T S Eliot
Four Quartets (Burnt Norton)

Only those are happy who never think.

E M Cioran
On the Heights of Despair

Life is a habit and the periods of transition represent the perilous zones in the life of the individual – dangerous, precarious, painful, mysterious, when for a moment the boredom of living is replaced by the suffering of being.

Samuel Beckett
Proust

You might imagine a heaven until you notice
The dull sad faces behind the coffee cups.

Roy Alexander
Coffee Bar

No matter where I start, I usually end up writing about pain…I set out to write about something lovely, like the diaphanous wing of a mayfly, and before long I find myself back in the shadows writing about the brief, tragic life of a mayfly.

How can I write about anything else?…Is there a more fundamental fact of human existence? I was born in pain…and I offered up, as my first evidence of life, a wail. I will likely die in pain as well. Between those brackets of pain I live out my days, limping from one towards the other. As…George Herbert put it, "I cried when I was born and every day shows why".

Philip Yancey
Soul Survivor

Pain, unlike pleasure, wears no mask. There are times when sorrow seems to me to be the only truth.

Oscar Wilde
De Profundis

O, that this too too solid flesh would melt,
Thaw, and resolve itself into a dew!
Or that the Everlasting had not fix'd
His canon 'gainst self-slaughter.

William Shakespeare
Hamlet

Don't look forward to the day you stop suffering, because when it comes, you're dead.

Tennessee Williams
The Observer, 1958

Have mercy upon me, O Lord, for I am in trouble: and mine eye is consumed for very heaviness; yea, my soul and my body.
For my life is waxen old with heaviness: and my years with mourning.

Psalm 31

"Please", you say, each in your own way, "take the pain away. Give me the magic pill or wave the magic wand or utter the magic formula and take the pain away".

Dorothy Rowe
Depression

Ever since I was born – that since has a resonance so dreadful to my ears it becomes unendurable.

E M Cioran
The Trouble With Being Born

To perceive is to suffer.

Aristotle
Unsourced

The conflict and tension between a desire to return to the whole, and to separate oneself from the collective is lifelong. We experience trauma at every point along life's journey: birth, weaning, toilet training, first steps, first day of school, leaving home, working out a meaningful vocation, marrying, loss of loved ones through death or rejection, and, ultimately our own deaths and illnesses and the physical limitations that presage them.

J L McNish
Cross Currents

My own heart let me more have pity on; let
Me live to my sad self hereafter kind,
Charitable; not live this tormented mind
With this tormented mind tormenting yet.
I cast for comfort I can no more get
By groping round my comfortless, than blind
Eyes in their dark can day or thirst can find
Thirst's all-in-all in all a world of wet.

Gerard Manley Hopkins
My Own Heart Let Me Have More Pity On

Happiness is but the occasional episode in a general drama of pain.

Thomas Hardy
The Mayor of Casterbridge

Life is not sweet. One day it will be sweet
To shut our eyes and die

Christina Rossetti
Life and Death

My appetite is lost; my nights are dreadful, and having nothing to do makes me dwell on past scenes...I would be glad if God took me. In the next world I could not be worse than I am in this.

Branwell Bronte
Letter to J B Leyland

I'm not afraid, 'cause no afterlife could ever suck as much as this one did.

Lyndon Morgans
Fairylights

No rose without a thorn. But many a thorn without a rose.

Arthur Schopenhauer
Essays and Aphorisms

The fact that man is never happy for the present is so true, that all his relief from unhappiness is only forgetting himself for a little while. Life is a progress from want to want, not from enjoyment to enjoyment.

Samuel Johnson
The Life of Samuel Johnson

We are never entirely free from pain at any stage in our life.

Peter Mullen
Death be not Proud

When we are born, we cry that we are come to this great stage of fools.

William Shakespeare
King Lear

Variable, and therefore miserable condition of Man; this minute I was well, and am ill, this minute.

John Donne
Devotion

Angel of gaiety, have you tasted grief?
Shame and remorse and sobs and weary spite,
And the vague terrors of the fearful night
That crush the heart up like a crumpled leaf?
Angel of kindness, have you tasted hate?
With hands clenched in the shade and tears of gall,
When Vengeance beats her hellish battle-call,
And makes herself the captain of our fate.

Angel of health, did you ever know pain,
Which like an exile trails his tired footfalls
The cold length of the white infirmary walls,
With lips compressed, seeking the sun in vain?

Angel of beauty, do you wrinkles know?
Know you the fear of age, the torment vile
Of reading secret horror in the smile
Of eyes your eyes have loved since long ago?

Charles Baudelaire
Reversibility

To each his sufferings: all are men
Condemned alike to groan.

Thomas Gray
Ode on a Distant Prospect of Eton College

Yes, indeed, there is more pain in life than gladness – it is one long agony until the grave.

Roubinovitch
La Melancolie

The syndrome known as life is too diffuse to admit of palliation. For every symptom that is eased, another is made worse.

Samuel Beckett
Murphy

Suffering is one very long moment. We cannot divide it by seasons. We can only record its moods, and chronicle their return. With us time itself does not progress. It revolves. It seems to circle round one centre of pain.

Oscar Wilde
De Profundis

For many a time
        I have been half in love with easeful Death,
Called him soft names in many a musèd rhyme,
To take into the air my quiet breath;
Now more than ever seems it rich to die,
To cease upon the midnight with no pain

John Keats
Ode to a Nightingale

It is silliness to live when to live is torment.

William Shakespeare
Othello

Hope is the worst of evils, for it prolongs the torments of man.

Friedrich Nietzsche
Human, All Too Human

Ah, woe is me for pleasure that is vain,
Ah, woe is me for glory that is past:
        Pleasure that bringeth sorrow at the last,
Glory that at the last bringeth no gain!
So saith the sinking heart; and so again
        It shall say till the mighty angel-blast
        Is blown, making the sun and moon aghast,
And showering down the stars like sudden rain.
And evermore men shall go fearfully
        Bending beneath their weight of heaviness;
And ancient men shall lie down wearily,
        And strong men shall rise up in weariness;
Yea, even the young shall answer sighingly
        Saying one to another: How vain it is!

Christina Rossetti
Vanity of Vanities

I groan within this tent of mine, being heavily burdened.
2 Corinthians V

To sensitive natures dismayed by life – and it seems that the four [Brontes]...were all, for different reasons, so dismayed – there is great comfort (and great danger) in the possession of an absorbing daydream in which to hide one's head.

Margaret Lane
The Bronte Story

Every scene of my life confirms the truth of what you have told me – there is no certain happiness in this state of being.

James Boswell
Letter to Samuel Johnson

This world is gradually becoming a place
Where I do not care to be any more.

John Berryman
The Dream Songs 149

Unhappy people are, in a sense, victims who suffer as they do on behalf of the rest of us an extreme of life's terrors and tensions.

Peter Mullen
Death be not Proud

The sense that every struggle brings defeat
        Because fate holds no prize to crown success;
That all the oracles are dumb or cheat
        Because they have no secret to express;
That none can pierce the vast black veil uncertain
Because there is no light behind the curtain;
        That all is vanity and nothingness.

James Thompson
The City of Dreadful Night

You have come into a hard world. I know of only one easy place in it, and that is the grave.

Henry Ward Beecher
Unsourced

Therefore is my spirit overwhelmed within me; my heart within me is desolate.

Psalm 142

All efforts to attain happiness are entirely futile.

E M Cioran
On the Heights of Despair

That she was not demonstratively thankful was no fault of hers. Her experience had been of a kind to teach her that the doubtful honour of a brief transit through a sorry world hardly called for effusiveness.

Thomas Hardy
The Mayor Of Casterbridge

Reality, looked at steadily, is unbearable.

C S Lewis
A Grief Observed

There is scarcely a draught of unmingled happiness to be had in this world.

Charlotte Bronte
The Life of Charlotte Bronte

Hard lot! Encompassed with a thousand dangers;
Weary, faint, trembling with a thousand terrors.

William Cowper
Lines Written During a Period of Insanity

For us there is only one season, the season of sorrow. The very sun and moon seem taken from us.

Oscar Wilde
De Profundis

Suffering is permanent, obscure, and dark
And has the nature of infinity.

William Wordsworth
The Borderers

Will fortune never come with both hands full,
But write her fair words still in foulest letters?
She either gives a stomach, and no food
Such are the poor, in health; or else a feast,
And takes away the stomach – such are the rich,
That have abundance, and enjoy it not.

William Shakespeare
Second Part of King Henry IV

I feel a nameless sadness o'er me roll.
Yes, yes, we know that we can jest,
We know, we know that we can smile!
But there's a something in this breast,
To which thy light words bring no rest.

Matthew Arnold
The Buried Life

In the healthiest and most prosperous existence, how many links of illness, danger, and disaster are always interposed? From the bottom of every fountain of pleasure, something bitter rises up: a touch of nausea, a falling dead of the delight, a whiff of melancholy, things that sound a knell, for fugitive as they may be, they bring a feeling of coming from a deeper region and often have an appalling convincingness. The buzz of life ceases at their touch as a piano-string stops sounding when the damper falls upon it.

William James
The Varieties of Religious Experience

And it never works out okay like in a movie.

Lyndon Morgans
Montparnasse

While affected with melancholy, all the doubts which have ever disturbed thinking men come upon me. I awake in the night dreading annihilation, or being thrown into some horrible state of being.

James Boswell
Boswell's Journal

Crying what I do is me: for that I came.

Gerard Manley Hopkins
Kingfishers Catch Fire

Nothing is more miserable than man,
Of all upon the earth that breathes and creeps.

Homer
Iliad

Many we are, and yet but few possess
Those fields of everlasting happiness.

Robert Herrick
Few Fortunate

Almost everyone I know is either overtly or covertly unhappy.

Chuck Klosterman
Sex, Drugs and Cocoa Puffs

We never taste happiness in perfection, our most fortunate successes are mixed with sadness.

Pierre Corneille
Unsourced

Melancholy is a fearful gift!
What is it but the telescope of truth?

George Gordon, Lord Byron
The Dream

So deep lie our sorrows, so deep in our souls!
So heavily, weigh down the fabric of life!
The struggling spirit is vanquished with strife,
Yet onward grief's torrent still merciless rolls

Colfax Burgoyne Harman
Sonnet to Sorrow

Even in laughter the heart is sorrowful; and the end of that mirth is heaviness.

Proverbs 14

Where is there an end of it, the soundless wailing,
The silent withering of autumn flowers...
        There is no end, but addition: the trailing
Consequence of further days and hours

T S Eliot
Four Quartets (The Dry Salvages)

It's like I've always lived in mourning,
Though for what I couldn't say.

Lyndon Morgans
I Bought a Rose From the Guy at the Traffic-Lights

Comfort's in heaven; and we are on the earth
Where nothing lives but crosses, care and grief.

William Shakespeare
Richard II

What are days for?
Days are where we live.
They come, they wake us
Time and time over.
They are to be happy in:
Where can we live but days?

Ah, solving that question
Brings the priest and the doctor
In their long coats
Running over the fields.

Philip Larkin
Days

Life's beastliness trampled me underfoot.

Emile Cioran
On the Heights of Despair

Vanity of vanities, the preacher saith
All things are vanity. The eye and ear
Cannot be filled with what they see and hear.
Like early dew, or like the sudden breath
Of wind, or like the grass that withereth
Is man, tossed to and fro by hope and fear,
So little joy has he, so little cheer,
Till all things end in the long dust of death.
Today is still the same as yesterday
Tomorrow also even as one of them,
And there is nothing new under the sun:
Until the ancient race of time be run
The old thorns shall grow out of the old stem
And morning shall be cold, and twilight grey.

Christina Rossetti
The One Certainty

What we gain by science is, after all, sadness. The more we know of the laws and nature of the Universe the more ghastly a business we perceive it all to be

Thomas Hardy
Unsourced

There is only one inborn erroneous notion…that we exist in order to be happy.

Arthur Schopenhauer
The World as Will and Representation

While many people discover tonics (…popularity, relationships, alcohol, drugs, religion…wealth) that appear to reduce the blatancy or effects of [the] intrinsic diseases [in us all], it seems as though we are all burned with an incurable mark of the plagues' existence within our souls.

Ashlyn Bradley
The Plague in All of Us

Fear, sickness, age, loss, labour, sorrow, strife,
Pain, hunger, cold that makes the heart to quake
And ever fickle fortune rageth rife
All which, and thousands more, do make a loathsome life.

Edmund Spenser
The Fairie Queene

The simple fact we must face is this: something is wrong with everything.

Larry Crabb
Inside Out

O happy shades! To me unblessed,
    Friendly to peace, but not to me!
How ill the scene that offers rest,
    And heart that cannot rest, agree!
This glassy stream, that spreading pine,
    Those alders quivering to the breeze,
Might sooth a soul less hurt than mine,
    And please, if anything could please.
But fixed unalterable Care
    Foregoes not what she feels within,
Shows the same sadness everywhere,
    And slights the season and the scene.

William Cowper
The Shrubbery

I am weary of groaning; every night wash I my bed: and water my couch with my tears.
My beauty is gone for very trouble: and I am worn away…

Psalm 6

Mankind is in a position similar to that of a set of people living on a frozen lake, surrounded by cliffs over which there is no escape, yet knowing that little by little the ice is melting, and the inevitable day drawing near when the last film of it will disappear, and to be drowned ignominiously will be the human creature's portion. The merrier the skating, the warmer and more sparkling the sun by day, and the ruddier the bonfires at night, the more poignant the sadness with which one must take in the meaning of the total situation.

William James
The Varieties of Religious Experience

Ah love, let us be true
To one another! for the world, which seems
To lie before us like a land of dreams,
So various, so beautiful, so new,
Hath really neither joy, nor love, nor light,
Nor certitude, nor peace, nor help for pain.

Matthew Arnold
Dover Beach

Now there's only one ambition left me; to die in my own bed.

Beverley Cross
Catherine Howard (TV episode)

Man that is born of a woman hath but a short time to live, and is full of misery. He cometh up, and is cut down, like a flower; he fleeth as it were a shadow and never continueth in one stay.

Book of Common Prayer

My thoughts hold mortal strife,
I do detest my life.

William Drummond
Madrigal

Eat, drink and play, and think that this is bliss
There is no Heaven but this!
There is no Hell;
Save Earth, which serves the purpose doubly well

Arthur Hugh Clough
Easter Day

Does the road wind uphill all the way?
    Yes, to the very end.

Christina Rossetti
Uphill

Of the demonstrably wise there are but two: those who commit suicide, and those who keep their reasoning faculties atrophied by drink.

Mark Twain
Note-Book

Tears always have deeper roots than smiles.

E M Cioran
On the Heights of Despair

[W]e are all divorced from life, we are all cripples, every one of us, more or less. We are so divorced from it that we feel…a sort of loathing for real life, and so cannot bear to be reminded of it…[W]e have come almost to looking upon real life as an effort, as hard work, and we are all privately agreed that it is better in books. Why [do we]…ask for something else? We don't know what ourselves. It would be the worse for us if our petulant prayers were answered.

Fyodor Dostoyevsky
Notes from the Underground

That I could clamber to the frozen moon
And draw the ladder after me.

Arthur Schopenhauer
Parerga and Paralipomena

Out of my nature has come wild despair; an abandonment to grief that was piteous even to look at; terrible and impotent rage; bitterness and scorn; anguish that wept aloud; misery that could find no voice; sorrow that was dumb.

Oscar Wilde
De Profundis

I don't know why we are here, but I'm pretty sure that it is not in order to enjoy ourselves.

Ludwig Wittgenstein

Quoted in *The Beginning of the End (2004)* by Peter Hershey

Optimism is cowardice.

Oswald Spengler
Man and Tactics

The sadness will last forever.

Vincent Van Gogh
(Last Words Of)

[L]ife for me is torture…

E M Cioran
On the Heights of Despair

I was just never much good at that happiness thing

Lyndon Morgans
The Time of Summer Lightning

Conclusion

Some people who know me thought that my purpose in compiling *The Agony Abides* was a pointless and destructive one, certainly as regards its effect on myself. One acquaintance said that even if I agreed with the quotations, there was no point in adding to my distress by immersing myself in such 'depressing stuff'.

I tried to explain that the 'depressing stuff' is actually not depressing at all. On the contrary, the quotations provide me with much needed solace in the midst of a life of often unmitigated gloom and despair. This is partly because they affirm my belief in the basic futility and joylessness of life and partly because they help me to know that I am not the only person to be dogged with a disconsolate disposition. As Jane Austen writes in *Persuasion*, "It is *singularity* which makes the worst part of our suffering..." (my italics).

If you have read and enjoyed this anthology, I assume you are a person who shares my melancholic mindset; someone who can understand what my friend Lyndon Morgans means when he speaks of having "always lived in mourning, though for what I couldn't say"[11]. As such a person, you will almost certainly have encountered admonitions to 'snap out of it', to 'look on the bright side' or to 'stop wallowing in self-pity'. These often well-intentioned comments aren't usually meant to be cruel, it's just that most people cannot comprehend the melancholic's conviction that life is, on the whole, little more than a tedious journey of wearisome pain.

When I first began compiling this anthology, my late father, (who was very much of an optimistic disposition!), read an early version of it, and though he commended me for the effort I had put into the work, he totally disagreed with its purpose and general ethos. Referring to Thomas Hardy's statement that "Happiness [is] but the occasional episode in a general drama of pain", my father said,

> 'You could equally state that pain is but the occasional episode in a general drama of happiness.'

You could. And I am sure it would be much pleasanter to be able to view life that way. But there are those amongst us who, with the best will in the world, cannot change our opinion that Thomas Hardy's statement is unfortunately, but indubitably, true.

In all sincerity I wish I could say that it wasn't. I wish that I could just enjoy the passages in my anthology in an artistic way, rather than believing and agreeing with what they say. But I can't. Like Lyndon, I *have* always "lived in mourning", and it isn't likely that, given the fact that the pains of life inevitably increase as we age and that my ethos has been proven and substantiated in numerous ways, I will ever change my long-held belief that life is a "dreary desert".

What I hope is that readers who share my sombre outlook on life have found some solace, consolation and even a sense of satisfaction that their beliefs have been validated. To all of you, I offer one piece of advice. Don't let *anybody* try to convince you that you are 'wrong'. You aren't. The poets, authors, philosophers and songwriters whose work is featured in my anthology are not abnormal, mentally ill or in need of counselling. On the contrary, they are highly intelligent, deep-feeling, profound-thinking people. But unfortunately it is such people who are usually far more disposed to suffer emotionally than are those of a more average intellect, shallow temperament and less acute sensitivity. As Ernest Hemingway said:

> "Happiness in intelligent people is the rarest thing I know."

No one who has read this anthology and, I hope, elicited some pleasure from the supremely talented writers whose quotations are featured in it, can doubt that he was right.

Bronwen Wrigley

Footnotes

1 C S Lewis, *The Problem of Pain*

2 Eric Fromm, *Brave New World Revisited* (Aldous Huxley)

3 Milan Kundera, *The Joke*

4 Oscar Wilde, *The Picture of Dorian Gray*

5 Voltaire, *Candide*

6 Malcolm Muggeridge, *Jesus Rediscovered*

7 James Thompson, *The City of Dreadful Night*

8 Dick Sullivan, *Poison Mixed With Gall, The Victorian Web*

9 Jesus said, "Are not five sparrows sold for two farthings, and not one of them is forgotten before God?" (Luke 12:6). Maybe not. But it doesn't stop them falling.

10 The reason why I have included this quotation is because the thought of a marriage which lasts for five decades deeply depresses me. The whole purpose of the comment in the TV programme was to emphasise how trapped married people often feel in a long marriage, and how stiflingly wearisome and dehumanising such a life can be.

11 Lyndon Morgans, *I Bought a Rose From the Guy at the Traffic-Lights*

Acknowledgements

I would like to thank the following for their kind permission to allow me to use copyright material

To David Higham Associates for use of extract from *Watership Down* by Richard Adams

To Faber and Faber for use of extracts from various works by Samuel Beckett

To Faber and Faber for use of extract from *Dream Song 149* by John Berryman

To Aitken Alexander Associates Ltd for use of extracts from various works by John Betjeman

To Curtis Brown Group Ltd., London on behalf of the Estate of Elizabeth Bowen Copyright (c) Elizabeth Bowen 1935 for use of extract from *The House in Paris* by Elizabeth Bowen

To Ashlyn Bradley for use of extracts from *The Plague in All of Us*

To Enitharmon Press for use of extract from *In This City* by Alan Brownjohn

To The Random House Group Ltd. for use of extract from *My Last Breath* by Luis Bunuel, published by Jonathan Cape

To SCM-Canterbury Press for use of extract from *The Coming of God* by Maria Boulding

To Curtis Brown Group Ltd, London on behalf of the estate of Beverley Cross Copyright Beverley Cross (c) 1970 and to the BBC for use of the extract taken from the episode 'Catherine Howard' from the TV Series *The Six Wives of Henry VIII*

To Curtis Brown Group Ltd, London on behalf of the Chichester Partnership Copyright (c) Daphne du Maurier 1938 for use of extract from *Rebecca*

To Jenny Brown Associates for use of extract from Introduction to *The Life of Samuel Johnson* by Angus Calder

To Hamish Hamilton (translator Joseph Laredo) for use of extract from *The Outsider* by Albert Camus

To Penguin Books (translator Robin Buss) for use of extract from *The Plague* by Albert Camus

To University of Chicago for use of extracts from *On the Heights of Despair* by E M Cioran

To Editions Gallimard for use of extracts from *The Trouble With Being Born* and *A Short History of Decay* by E M Cioran

To Roy Clarke and SD-Office and the BBC for use of extracts from the TV Series *Last of the Summer Wine* by Roy Clarke

To Simon and Schuster for use of the extract from *Life After God* by Douglas Coupland

To NavPress for permission to use extracts from *Inside Out* by Larry Crabb

To John Daulman for use of his two extracts

To Princeton University Press for use of extracts from *Pessimism: Philosophy, Ethic, Spirit* by Joshua Foa Dienstag

To Faber and Faber Ltd. for use of extracts from several works by T S Eliot in *Collected Poems 1909-1962* by T S Eliot

To David Higham for use of extract from *The Great Gatsby* by F Scott Fitzgerald

To The Random House Group Ltd for use of extract from *The City People Meet Themselves* by Roseanne Flynn from Wondercrump Poetry edited by Jennifer Curry, published by Red Fox

To Aitken Alexander Associates Ltd for use of extract from *The Collector* by John Fowles

To Pink Floyd Music Publishers Ltd for use of lyric from *Poles Apart* by David Gilmour

To Winston Graham (Copyright © Winston Graham) reprinted by permission of A M Heath & Co Ltd for use of extracts from *Demelza*, *Jeremy Poldark* and *Ross Poldark*

To David Higham and Vintage for use of extract from *The Heart of the Matter* by Graham Greene

To Graham Wrench for use of lyrics from *Lady's Bridge* by Richard Hawley

To Century for use of extract from *Into the Forest* by Jean Hegland, reprinted by permission of The Random House Group Ltd.

To Penguin Books for use of extract from *The Garden of Eden* by Ernest Hemingway

To Mike Hugg and Ian la Frenais for use of extracts from the lyrics from the film *The Likely Lads* and the BBC TV Series *Whatever Happened to the Likely Lads*

To Darton, Longman and Todd Ltd and Eerdmans Publishing Co, for use of extract from *God of Surprises* by Gerard Hughes

To Crescent Moon Publishing for use of extract from *In the Still Void* by Gregory Johns

To Faber and Faber for use of extract from *Sex, Drugs and Cocoa Puffs* by Chuck Klosterman

To St. Anthony Messenger Press, 28 W Liberty St, Cincinnati, OH 45202 for use of extracts from *Making Sense Out of Suffering* by Peter Kreeft copyright 1986. To order copies visit www.servantbooks.org

To Berlin Associates for use of extracts from *I Dreamed a Dream* by Herbert Kretzmer

To George Landow for use of extract from The Victorian Website

To Selina Hastings for use of extracts from *The Bronte Story* by Margaret Lane

To C. S. Lewis copyright (c) C S Lewis Pte Ltd 1933 for use of extracts from *Pilgrim's Regress*

To Faber and Faber for use of extracts from works by Philip Larkin in *Collected Poems* by Philip Larkin

To Faber and Faber for use of extracts from *A Grief Observed* by C S Lewis

To Archie Bevan, literary executor for The Estate of George Mackay Brown for use of extract from *First Fall* by George Mackay Brown

To David Higham Associates for the use of extracts from *Espresso Tales* (Polygon 2005) and *44 Scotland Street* (Polygon 2005) by Alexander McCall Smith

To EMI Music Publishing Ltd for lyrics by Paddy McAloon

To Charles Henderson, Cross Currents for use of extract from *Cross Currents* by J L McNish

To Enoch Pratt Free Library, Baltimore for use of extracts from *Chrestomathy* and by H L Mencken

To Curtis Brown for use of extract from *Black Spring* by Henry Miller

To Lyndon Morgans for use of lyrics from all his songs

To Peter Mullen for use of extracts from *The New Babel* and *Death Be Not Proud*

Extract from *The Examined Life* by Robert Nozick, copyright (c) 1989 by Robert Nozick, reprinted by permission of Georges Borchardt Inc., on behalf of the Estate of Robert Nozick

To The London Library for use of the extract from *Afterthoughts* by Logan Pearsall-Smith

To Faber and Faber for use of extracts from *Monogamy* by Adam Phillips

To Faber and Faber for use of extracts from works by Ezra Pound in *Collected Poems* by Ezra Pound

To Mark Green of M Green Production for use of lyrics from *I Was Right* by Ricky Ross Ricky

To Aitken Alexander Associates for use of extracts from *Depression* by Dorothy Rowe

To Peters, Fraser and Dunlop and to the BBC for use of extract from BBC TV Series *Poldark*

To the Estate of George Sassoon for use of extract from *Everyman* by Siegfried Sassoon

To the estate of Vernon Scannell for use of the poem *Where Shall We Go?*

To Free Methodist Communications for use of extract from *Healing Grace* by David Seamands

To executors of James MacGibbon for use of *Not Waving But Drowning* by Stevie Smith

To Constant Artists for use of lyrics from all songs by Will Sheff

To The Literary Estate of Arthur Symons for use of his poem *At Dawn*

To Emmett Tinley for use of lyrics from all his songs

To Wiley-Blackwell for use of extract from *No Alternative* by Rachel Trickett

To Mark Fenwick for use of lyrics from all songs by Roger Waters

To the Master and Fellows of Trinity College Cambridge for use of extract from *Beginning of the End* by Ludwig Wittgenstein

To Georges Borchardt Lnc on behalf of the University of the South for use of extracts from works by Tennessee Williams: *Orpheus Descending*, copyright (c) 1955, 1958 by Tennessee Williams

The Rose Tattoo, copyright (c) 1950, 1951 by Tennessee Williams.

The Milk Train Doesn't Stop Here Anymore, copyright (c) 1976 by Tennessee Williams

from *The London Observer*, copyright 1958 by Tennessee Williams

To Charlotte Wrigley for use of extract from *The Vagabond*

To Hodder & Stoughton, Hodder Faith, Headline Publishing Group and John Murray (Publishers) for use of extract from *Soul Survivor* by Philip Yancey